Hematologic Issues in Critical Care

Editor

PATRICIA O'MALLEY

CRITICAL CARE NURSING CLINICS OF NORTH AMERICA

www.ccnursing.theclinics.com

Consulting Editor
JAN FOSTER

September 2017 • Volume 29 • Number 3

ELSEVIER

1600 John F. Kennedy Boulevard • Suite 1800 • Philadelphia, Pennsylvania, 19103-2899

http://www.theclinics.com

CRITICAL CARE NURSING CLINICS OF NORTH AMERICA Volume 29, Number 3
September 2017 ISSN 0899-5885, ISBN-13: 978-0-323-54548-8

Editor: Kerry Holland
Developmental Editor: Colleen Dietzler

Critical Care Nursing Clinics of North America (ISSN 0899-5885) is published quarterly by Elsevier Inc., 360 Park Avenue South, New York, NY 10010-1710. Months of issue are March, June, September, and December. Business and Editorial Offices: 1600 John F. Kennedy Blvd., Suite 1800, Philadelphia, PA 19103-2899. Periodicals postage paid at New York, NY and additional mailing offices. Subscription prices are $155.00 per year for US individuals, $385.00 per year for US institutions, $100.00 per year for US students and residents, $200.00 per year for Canadian individuals, $483.00 per year for Canadian institutions, $230.00 per year for international individuals, $483.00 per year for international institutions and $115.00 per year for Canadian and international students/residents. To receive student/resident rate, orders must be accompanied by name of affiliated institution, data of term, and the *signature* of program/residency coordinator on institution letterhead. Orders will be billed at individual rate until proof of status is received. Foreign air speed delivery is included in all *Clinics* subscription prices. All prices are subject to change without notice. **POSTMASTER:** Send address changes to *Critical Care Nursing Clinics of North America*, Elsevier Health Sciences Division, Subscription Customer Service, 3251 Riverport Lane, Maryland Heights, MO 63043. **Customer Service: 1-800-654-2452 (US and Canada); 314-447-8871 (outside US and Canada). Fax: 314-447-8029. E-mail:** JournalsCustomerService-usa@elsevier.com **(for print support) and** JournalsOnlineSupport-usa@elsevier.com **(for online support).**

Reprints. For copies of 100 or more of articles in this publication, please contact the Commercial Reprints Department, Elsevier Inc., 360 Park Avenue South, New York, New York, 10010-1710; Tel.: 212-633-3874, Fax: 212-633-3820, and E-mail: reprints@elsevier.com.

Critical Care Nursing Clinics of North America is covered in *MEDLINE/PubMed (Index Medicus), International Nursing Index, Nursing Citation Index, Cumulative Index to Nursing and Allied Health Literature, and RNdex Top 100.*

Contributors

CONSULTING EDITOR

JAN FOSTER, PhD, APRN, CNS
Formerly, Associate Professor, College of Nursing, Texas Woman's University, Houston, Texas; President, Nursing Inquiry and Intervention, Inc, The Woodlands, Texas

EDITOR

PATRICIA O'MALLEY, PhD, RN, APRN-CNS
Nurse Researcher/Faculty, Department of Nursing Research, Premier Health, Center of Nursing Excellence, Dayton, Ohio; Adjunct Faculty, School of Nursing, Indiana University East, Richmond, Indiana

AUTHORS

MARIE BASHAW, DNP, RN, NEA-BC
Assistant Professor, College of Nursing and Health, Wright State University, Dayton, Ohio

TONYA BREYMIER, PhD, RN, CNE, COI
Associate Dean and Assistant Professor, School of Nursing and Health Sciences, Indiana University East, Richmond, Indiana

MICHELLE R. BROWN, MS, MLS (ASCP)^{CM}SBB^{CM}
Assistant Professor, Clinical Laboratory Science, University of Alabama at Birmingham, Birmingham, Alabama

ANDREW BUGAJSKI, BSN, RN
Doctoral Student, College of Nursing, University of Kentucky, Lexington, Kentucky

CHARLES C. CALDWELL, PhD
Division of Research, Department of Surgery, College of Medicine, University of Cincinnati, Cincinnati, Ohio

SUSAN K. FRAZIER, PhD, RN, FAHA
Associate Professor and Director, PhD Program, Co-director, RICH Heart Program, College of Nursing, University of Kentucky, Lexington, Kentucky

JACOB HIGGINS, BSN, RN
Doctoral Student, College of Nursing, University of Kentucky, Lexington, Kentucky

ALLISON R. JONES, PhD, RN, CCNS
Assistant Professor, Department of Acute, Chronic and Continuing Care, School of Nursing, University of Alabama at Birmingham, Birmingham, Alabama

BETSY BABB KENNEDY, PhD, RN, CNE
Associate Professor, Director of Faculty Development, Vanderbilt University School of Nursing, Nashville, Tennessee

JARED MANDOZA, BSN, RN
Department of Nursing, College of Nursing and Health Sciences, University of Wisconsin–Eau Claire, Eau Claire, Wisconsin

BRIANNE MANSFIELD, DNP, RN, APRN, NP-C
Nurse Practitioner, Radiation Oncology, Mayo Clinic, Rochester, Minnesota

KELLY McCOY, BSN, RN
Coordinator, Blood Management, Cleveland Clinic Health System, Cleveland, Ohio

SUZANNE McMURTRY BAIRD, DNP, RN
President, Clinical Concepts in Obstetrics, Inc, Staff Nurse, Labor and Delivery, Vanderbilt University Medical Center, Adjunct Faculty, Vanderbilt University School of Nursing, Nashville, Tennessee

PATRICIA O'MALLEY, PhD, RN, APRN-CNS
Nurse Researcher/Faculty, Department of Nursing Research, Premier Health, Center of Nursing Excellence, Dayton, Ohio; Adjunct Faculty, School of Nursing, Indiana University East, Richmond, Indiana

JANET L. PETTY, MLIS, AHIP
System Coordinator, Patient and Family Education, Premier Health Learning Institute, Craig Memorial Library, Miami Valley Hospital, Dayton, Ohio

AMANDA M. PUGH, MD
Division of Research, Department of Surgery, College of Medicine, University of Cincinnati, Cincinnati, Ohio

DEBORAH A. RAINES, PhD, EDS, RN, ANEF
Associate Professor, School of Nursing, University at Buffalo, Buffalo, New York

TERESA C. RICE, MD
Division of Research, Department of Surgery, College of Medicine, University of Cincinnati, Cincinnati, Ohio

TONYA RUTHERFORD-HEMMING, EdD, RN, ANP-BC, CHSE
Clinical Associate Professor, School of Nursing, University of North Carolina at Greensboro, Greensboro, North Carolina

SHIRLEY SEBALD-KINDER, MLS, AHIP
Manager, Premier Health Learning Institute, Craig Memorial Library, Miami Valley Hospital, Dayton, Ohio

BARBARA ST. PIERRE SCHNEIDER, PhD, RN
Research Professor of Nursing, The Tony and Renee Marlon Angel Network Professorship, School of Nursing, University of Nevada, Las Vegas, Las Vegas, Nevada

DOUGLAS H. SUTTON, EdD, MSN, MPA, APRN, NP-C
Associate Professor, College of Health and Human Services, Northern Arizona University, Flagstaff, Arizona

DEBORAH J. TOLICH, DNP, RN
Director, Blood Management, Cleveland Clinic Health System, Cleveland, Ohio

LINDA K. YOUNG, PhD, RN, CNE, CFLE
Dean, Department of Nursing, College of Nursing and Health Sciences, University of Wisconsin–Eau Claire, Eau Claire, Wisconsin

Contents

Transfusion, a common practice in critical care, is not without complication. Acute adverse reactions to transfusion occur within 24 hours and
include acute hemolytic transfusion reaction, febrile nonhemolytic transfusion reaction, allergic and anaphylactic reactions, and transfusion-related
acute lung injury, transfusion-related infection or sepsis, and transfusion-
associated circulatory overload. Delayed transfusion adverse reactions
develop 48 hours or more after transfusion and include erythrocyte and
platelet alloimmunization, delayed hemolytic transfusion reactions, post-
transfusion purpura, transfusion-related immunomodulation, transfusion-
associated graft versus host disease, and, with long-term transfusion,
iron overload. Clinical strategies may reduce the likelihood of reactions
and improve patient outcomes.

This article reviews treatments and strategies that can be used to reduce,
or as adjuncts to, blood transfusion to manage blood volumes in patients
who are critically ill. Areas addressed include iatrogenic anemia, fluid management, pharmaceutical agents, hemostatic agents, hemoglobin-based
oxygen carriers, and management of patients for whom blood is not an
option.

This systematic literature review informs the clinician caring for the critically ill patient of the risks associated with red blood cell (RBC) transfusion.
Data were extracted from publications between 2008 and 2016 and were
reviewed to determine their usefulness in providing evidence associated
with the risk of receiving an RBC transfusion. They reveal that this intervention may exacerbate certain clinical conditions and increase mortality and
morbidity rates. Further scientific study is needed to better inform clinical
practitioners about the inherent risks and benefits associated with the
common clinical intervention of RBC transfusion in the critically ill patient.

folate, and vitamin B_{12}, which will reduce risks associated with blood transfusions.

Simulation has emerged in health care education programs over the past few decades. Acute-care institutions now provide simulation and high-fidelity simulation (HFS) experiences, nurse development, competency training, and evaluation. The International Association for Clinical Simulation and Learning has established best practice guidelines and a framework for multiple skills, such as blood transfusion. The Institute of Medicine report, *To Err Is Human*, brought patient safety issues to the forefront. Blood transfusion management is a skill for which HFS can provide a safe environment to educate and evaluate nurse competencies for blood transfusion management processes.

Searching the literature can be challenging because of the large volume of information. It can be time consuming to locate and determine what evidence will provide the best health outcomes for patients. In addition, locating hematology information for patients and family members is one of the most challenging of all health care topics. Hematology can be technical and difficult for most people to understand, especially for those with little or no science background and poor reading skills. This article provides guidance on how and where to locate information to address the needs of both clinicians and patients.

This article explores anemia without an obvious cause from two perspectives: a patient and the evidence. Although evidence is required to drive favorable patient outcomes, the focus on evidence often hides the patient experience during diagnosis and treatment. Knowledge of experience with evidence can provide a deeper perspective for clinical decision making and meet nursing's ethical mandate to relieve suffering. Although one patient experience does not reflect every patient experience, this patient's experience demonstrates how difficult and dark anemia can be.

CRITICAL CARE NURSING
CLINICS OF NORTH AMERICA

ISSUE OF RELATED INTEREST

Hematology/Oncology Clinics, June 2016 (Vol. 30, Issue 3)
Transfusion Medicine
Jeanne E. Hendrickson and Christopher A. Tormey, *Editors*
Available at: http://www.hemonc.theclinics.com

THE CLINICS ARE AVAILABLE ONLINE!
Access your subscription at:
www.theclinics.com

Preface

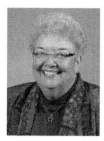

Patricia O'Malley, PhD, RN, APRN-CNS
Editor

Imbedded throughout the critical illness landscape is blood. A core element of life and death, violence and war, families and donors, sacrifice and spirit, blood is life sustaining and lifesaving.

Critical care nursing practice is impacted by blood in every way. Nurses monitor blood, infuse blood, and manage blood to preserve oxygenation, waste removal, organ function, and nutrient delivery. As a result, immunity, hormone transport, pH balance, and body temperature regulation are also sustained.

This issue of *Critical Care Nursing Clinics of North America* provides the reader evidence and best practices for common as well as emerging hematologic issues in critical care nursing practice. Dr Frazier provides the reader with current best practices for blood management in the intensive care unit (ICU). Alternatives for blood replacement in the ICU are investigated by Dr Tolich. The risks associated with just one unit of blood are explored for practice by Dr Sutton.

Some of the most difficult hematologic issues in the ICU are also charted. Dr Kennedy provides current best practices for the management of obstetric hemorrhage. Blood transfusion in sepsis and the relationship to proinflammatory and counterinflammatory immune responses are examined by Dr Schneider. Dr Young provides much needed direction on nursing care for the bone marrow and blood cell transplant patient in the ICU. Finally, I explore the hidden anemias in the critically ill related to drug therapies and disease. I believe you will be as surprised as I was by how much hidden anemia there is.

No review of hematologic issues in the ICU would be complete without a current examination of coagulopathy in and outside the ICU, which Dr Bashaw provides. For practice and education, Dr Breymier provides a valuable analysis regarding the use of high-fidelity simulation to increase knowledge and skills to care for patients receiving blood products. Finally, Sebald-Kinder and Petty provide the reader with a treasure of hematologic resources for practice, education, and research.

To balance this issue of evidence and best practices, a short case study is provided for reflection and perspective. May this article, "The Lived Experience of Anemia

Crit Care Nurs Clin N Am 29 (2017) ix–x
http://dx.doi.org/10.1016/j.cnc.2017.06.001
0899-5885/17/© 2017 Published by Elsevier Inc.

ccnursing.theclinics.com

Without a Cause," provide a foundation for a critical eye to recognize earlier rather than later the insidious effects of anemia on body, mind, and spirit.

Patricia O'Malley, PhD, RN, APRN-CNS
Department of Nursing Research
Premier Health
Center of Nursing Excellence
1 Wyoming Street
Dayton, OH 45409, USA

School of Nursing
Indiana University East
2325 Chester Boulevard
Richmond, IN 47374, USA

E-mail address:
pomalley@premierhealth.com

Adverse Reactions to Transfusion of Blood Products and Best Practices for Prevention

Susan K. Frazier, PhD, RN[a],*, Jacob Higgins, BSN, RN[b],
Andrew Bugajski, BSN, RN[b], Allison R. Jones, PhD, RN, CCNS[c],
Michelle R. Brown, MS, MLS (ASCP)[CM]SBB[CM][d]

KEYWORDS

- Blood components • Transfusion • Adverse transfusion reactions • TACO • TRALI
- Restrictive transfusion strategy

KEY POINTS

- Acute adverse reactions to transfusion occur within 24 hours and may be immune or non-immune in origin; most occur within 4 hours of transfusion. Delayed reactions occur 48 hours or more after transfusion and are primarily immune in origin.
- Strategies currently used to reduce adverse transfusion reactions include donor and donated blood screening, leukoreduction, irradiation, premedication with acetaminophen, diphenhydramine, and furosemide, restrictive transfusion protocols, cell salvage and autotransfusion, and devices and practices to reduce iatrogenic anemia, although research evidence is not supportive of several of these strategies.
- The use of restrictive transfusion protocols with a transfusion trigger hemoglobin of 8 g/dL for orthopedic and cardiac surgery patients is supported with high-quality evidence.

INTRODUCTION

Annually, nearly 14 million units of whole blood and packed red cells (PRC) are transfused worldwide; in the United States, approximately 36,000 units of PRC, 7000 units of platelets, and 10,000 units of fresh frozen plasma (FFP) are transfused each year.[1]

The authors have nothing to disclose.
[a] PhD Program, RICH Heart Program, College of Nursing, University of Kentucky, CON Building, Office 523, 751 Rose Street, Lexington, KY 40536-0232, USA; [b] College of Nursing, University of Kentucky, CON Building, 751 Rose Street, Lexington, KY 40536-0232, USA; [c] Department of Acute, Chronic & Continuing Care, School of Nursing, University of Alabama at Birmingham, NB 543, 1720 2nd Avenue South, Birmingham, AL 35294-1210, USA; [d] Clinical Laboratory Science, University of Alabama at Birmingham, SHPB 474, 1705 University Boulevard, Birmingham, AL 35294, USA
* Corresponding author.
E-mail address: skfraz2@email.uky.edu

Crit Care Nurs Clin N Am 29 (2017) 271–290
http://dx.doi.org/10.1016/j.cnc.2017.04.002

Transfusion of blood products in critical care is common; scientists estimated that 15% to 53% of critically ill patients are transfused during their critical care stay.[2] Blood transfusion in the intensive care unit is primarily used to increase oxygen-carrying capacity reduced by anemia. Anemia in the critical care unit is multifactorial and may be associated with nutritional deficiencies of iron, folate or vitamin B, cell hemolysis, coagulopathies, erythropoietin deficiencies, and blood loss due to trauma, surgery, hemorrhage, or iatrogenic reason.[3,4] Although transfusion is a common practice in the critical care unit, it is not without complication.

Recently, scientists analyzed 125 data sets representing 25 countries from the International Haemovigilance Network Database and determined the rate of adverse reactions to transfusion of blood products was 660 per 100,000 individuals; nearly 3% of these were categorized as severe.[5] The mortality associated with transfusion was 0.26 deaths per 100,000; nearly 60% of deaths were due to transfusion-associated circulatory overload (TACO), transfusion-related lung injury (TRALI), and transfusion-associated dyspnea (TAD). Harvey and colleagues[6] analyzed transfusion data from 77 facilities in the United States and found that there were 239.5 adverse reactions per 100,000 units transfused. Allergic reactions were the most common type with 112.2 reactions per 100,000 units transfused. Severe adverse reactions occurred at a rate of 17.5 per 100,000 units transfused. Platelet transfusion had the highest rate at 421.7 per 100,000 units; rates for PRC, plasma, and cryoprecipitate were 205.5, 127.7, and 5.6 per 100,000 units, respectively. Although transfusion of blood components is common, adverse reactions to those transfusions may produce mild to severe adverse reactions.

HISTORICAL CONTEXT

Although references to blood transfusion can be found as early as 32 BC in early Greek and Roman myths, these likely referred to drinking blood rather than actual transfusion as we understand it. In 1612, William Harvey described the circulatory system, and subsequently, a variety of scientists described and attempted transfusions, primarily in animals. In the early 1800s, Dr James Blundell performed the first reported human to human transfusions; the first successful transfusion was from his assistant to a woman with postpartum hemorrhage.[7,8] However, some early attempts transfused blood from cadavers to live patients for treatment of various illnesses.[9]

In 1900, Landsteiner and other scientists described 4 blood types and subsequently proposed a classification system for international use; this system was universally adopted in the 1950s.[10] With the need for treatment of patients after war trauma during World War II, direct whole blood transfusions was replaced with component transfusion once science developed techniques for separation of whole blood and storage of components.[9] However, reports of recipient hepatitis after transfusion eventually led to the initiation of screening donor blood for infectious diseases.[11] In addition to infectious transmission, multiple adverse reactions were observed and described over the past 200 years; in fact, Dr Blundell reported several adverse reactions with his initial person-to-person transfusions.[7] Researchers and clinicians are now aware of multiple adverse reactions that may occur; recent data demonstrated that TRALI and TACO accounted for 38% and 24%, respectively, of transfusion-associated fatalities from 2011 to 2015.[12]

ADVERSE REACTIONS TO TRANSFUSION OF BLOOD PRODUCTS
Acute Reactions

Acute adverse reactions to transfusion are those that occur within 24 hours; however, most occur within 4 hours of transfusion[13] (**Table 1**). Acute reactions may be immune

Table 1
Acute adverse transfusion reactions

Reaction	Signs and Symptoms	Management
AHTR	Fever, chills, dyspnea, hypotension, hemoglobinuria, chest or flank pain, nausea and vomiting, oliguria/anuria, disseminated intravascular coagulation (DIC), positive direct anti-globulin test (DAT) for IgG and/or complement	Furosemide and fluid administration to remove free hemoglobin and reduce likelihood of acute renal failure, symptomatic treatment of anemia, hypotension, and DIC, transfusion of blood components
FNHTR	Within 4 h of transfusion core temperature of 100.4°F (38°C) or an increase of 1.8°F (1°C) from the pretransfusion value with or without chills and rigor	Symptom management: antipyretic Narcotic for chills and rigor For subsequent transfusion: leukoreduction, washed PRCs
Allergic and anaphylactic transfusion reactions	Mild, pruritis, urticaria Anaphylactic, angioedema, bronchoconstriction, stridor, hypotension, wheezing, tachycardia	Mild, antihistamine Anaphylactic: epinephrine, corticosteroids, antihistamine, fluid bolus
TRALI	Within 6 h of transfusion: $Pao_2/Fio_2 \leq 300$ or $SaO_2 \leq 90\%$ Bilateral pulmonary infiltrates Dyspnea, cyanosis, hypoxemia, hypotension	Oxygen therapy, intubation and mechanical ventilation as required Vasopressors as indicated, symptomatic support

Transfusion-transmitted infections	Bacterial: Fever of 102°F or >3.6°F increase from pretransfusion, rigor, chills, tachycardia, backache, abdominal pain, vomiting, and hypothermia
	Viral: seroconversion
	  In immunocompromised individuals, West Nile virus may develop meningoencephalitis
	  With HTLV-1, myelopathy with spastic paraparesis, adult T-cell leukemia/lymphoma
	Protozoal infections:
	  Plasmodium species: malaria
	  Trypanosoma cruzi: Chagas disease
	  Babesia microti: malaria-like illness
	  Leishmania donovani: leishmaniasis
	Prion disease
	  Human bovine spongiform encephalopathy, variant Creutzfeldt-Jacob disease
		Stop transfusion, culture the transfused unit, and draw blood cultures, empiric antibiotics
		Prevention by systematic donor screening for exposure to viruses, testing of donated blood, symptomatic therapy, potentially therapy for HepB
		Malaria
		  Dependent on species, chloroquinine, atovaquone-proguanil, artemether-lumefantrine, mefloquine, quinine, quinidine, doxycycline with quinine, clindamycin quinine
		Chagas
		  Benznidazole or nifurtimox
		Leishmaniasis
		  Sodium stibogluconate available in United States only from the Centers for Disease Control and Prevention, for cutaneous, mucosal and visceral, miltefosine, for visceral, intravenous liposomal amphotericin B
		Currently no treatment

(continued on next page)

Table 1 (continued)		
Reaction	**Signs and Symptoms**	**Management**
TACO	Within 1–2 h of transfusion dyspnea, orthopnea, cyanosis, cough, hypoxemia, hypertension, hydrostatic pulmonary edema, B-type or brain natriuretic peptide concentration >100 pg/mL	Slow transfusion, reduce fluid intake, oxygen therapy, diuretics, afterload reduction

Data from Dasararaju R, Marques MB. Adverse effects of transfusion. Cancer Control. 2015;22(1):16–25; and American Association of Blood Banks. Circular of information for the use of human blood and blood components. 2016. Available at: https://www.aabb.org/tm/coi/Documents/coi1113.pdf.

or nonimmune in origin. Immune adverse reactions typically occur in response to antigens on the transfused erythrocytes or leukocytes, platelets, or plasma proteins. These reactions include acute hemolytic transfusion reaction (AHTR), febrile nonhemolytic transfusion reaction (FNHTR), allergic and anaphylactic reactions, and TRALI. Nonimmune reactions include transfusion-related infection or sepsis, and TACO. TAD, acute dyspnea within 24 hours of transfusion, is diagnosed when patient symptoms are not related to the existing diagnoses, and the criteria for allergic reaction, TRALI, and TACO are not met (see **Table 1**).[14,15]

Acute hemolytic transfusion reaction

Between 2011 and 2015, there were 37 fatal hemolytic transfusion reactions reported to the US Food and Drug Administration (FDA); 7.5% were due to ABO incompatibility.[12] Hemolytic transfusion reactions produce rapid, accelerated erythrocyte destruction because of interaction between antigens on the donor erythrocytes and recipient antibodies, or antigens on recipient erythrocytes and antibodies in the donor plasma.[16] Antibodies in these reactions are typically from the immunoglobulin M (IgM) class of antibodies, and the reaction may be extravascular or intravascular.[17] With intravascular hemolysis, 200 mL of erythrocytes can be hemolyzed in 1 hour, and total hemoglobin can be reduced by 5 g in a few hours.

The consequence of intravascular erythrocyte destruction is the release of free hemoglobin, which in circulation will be bound to plasma proteins, haptoglobin, hemopexin, and albumin.[17] Once these plasma proteins are saturated, free hemoglobin is filtered in the glomerulus and may be reabsorbed, or excreted in the urine when the reabsorption capacity of the tubule is exceeded. With complete complement activation, mast cells are also stimulated to release histamine and serotonin; the result is vasodilation, plasma leak from the vascular endothelial wall, third spacing of vascular fluid, and subsequent hypotension. In addition, cytokine release from leukocytes is stimulated by hemolysis, and a systemic inflammatory response syndrome is the consequence, with subsequent fever, hypotension, activation of neutrophils, induction of adhesion molecules, and endothelial damage.[15] Simultaneous activation of the kallikrein-kinin system and the coagulation cascade further increases capillary permeability, produces arteriolar dilation, and disseminated intravascular coagulation with diffuse microcirculatory coagulation. Consumption of coagulation factors and diffuse bleeding are the consequence. Multiple organ dysfunction and eventual organ failure may ensue.

Febrile nonhemolytic transfusion reaction

Nonhemolytic transfusion reaction is the most common transfusion-associated adverse event with prevalence as high as 60% of all adverse reactions.[13,18] Within 4 hours of transfusion, individuals develop fever (increase from pretransfusion temperature of 1.8°F or 1°C) with or without chills; other possible symptoms include nausea and vomiting, dyspnea, and non-life-threatening hypotension.[19] Symptoms are usually self-limiting, but the risk for recurrence with subsequent transfusion is 15%.[20] FNHTRs are caused by transfusion of proinflammatory cytokines accumulated during component storage, and the interaction of recipient antibodies and human leukocyte antigen or leukocyte-specific antigens on donor leukocytes.[15,19]

Proinflammatory cytokine concentration is associated with storage time. The longer the storage time, the higher the concentration of proinflammatory cytokines; prestorage leukoreduction of components does reduce this effect by as much as 50%.[21,22] The likelihood for FNHTR increases as the number of transfused units increases; in individuals 65 years of age and older, odds of an FNHTR were 15% and 25% higher with female sex and prior transfusion within the previous year.[23]

Allergic and anaphylactic transfusion reactions

Minor allergic transfusion reactions occur in as many as 31% of critical care patients[13]; however, mortality from anaphylaxis was reported to be only 5% of all reactions in the period from 2011 to 2015.[12] Thus, allergic reactions are common, but anaphylactic reactions rare. Allergic reactions are commonly associated with urticaria, flushing, and pruritis.[15] Allergic reactions are typically IgE-mediated type 1 hypersensitivity reactions. Activation of mast cells and basophils produces release of inflammatory mediators like histamine, leukotriene, and prostaglandin; complement activation and proinflammatory cytokines released from macrophages also contribute to this type of reaction. Transfusion recipients react to an immunologically active compound in the transfused blood component; the recipient has previously been sensitized to this compound. The actual stimulus for the reaction is typically unknown, but may include plasma proteins like haptoglobin, complement and albumin, and chemicals that may include drugs ingested by the donor before donation.[24,25] Food allergens in the donor blood have also been hypothesized to produce allergic transfusion reactions, but there are no data currently to support this hypothesis.[26]

Although rare, anaphylactic transfusion reactions may be deadly; these are caused by recipient antibodies to donor plasma proteins. Symptoms are those of anaphylaxis and include angioedema, stridor, respiratory distress, and bronchoconstriction with dyspnea and wheezing. Histamine also produces vasodilation and significant decrease in systemic vascular resistance with subsequent hypotension. This type of reaction requires systematic investigation to ensure that the individual is not exposed to the immunologically active culprit again in future transfusions. The use of newer platelet additive solutions for platelet transfusions replaces most of the plasma and reduced the allergic reactions with this component by nearly one third.[27]

Transfusion-related acute lung injury

TRALI is new onset, acute lung injury that is evidenced within 6 hours of transfusion. Signs include bilateral pulmonary infiltrates without left atrial enlargement, Pao_2/Fio_2 of 300 mm Hg or less and SpO_2 90% or less, absence of acute lung injury before transfusion, and absence of other alternative risk factors.[28] TRALI is the primary cause of transfusion-associated mortality; 38% of reported deaths related to transfusion were due to TRALI.[12] TRALI occurs when antibodies to human leukocyte and/or human neutrophil antigens are present in transfused components.[29] In response, neutrophils are sequestered in pulmonary tissue and become activated following sequestration. TRALI may also result from transfusion of biologically activated lipids or cytokines; these may also stimulate neutrophils and produce TRALI. Neutrophils also accumulate in other organs and subsequently produce organ damage, dysfunction, and failure. Clinically, TRALI is not distinguishable from acute respiratory disease syndrome (ARDS); however, TRALI may be associated with acute neutropenia, and human neutrophil antibodies were found in 22% to 42% of cases.[15,29] With supportive management, most individuals recover oxygenation ability in 48 to 96 hours; however, mortality from TRALI is reported to range from 5% to 25%.[15]

Transfusion-transmitted infections

Transfusion of infected blood components may transmit gram-negative and -positive bacteria, viruses, protozoa, and prions to the recipient. Although surveillance has identified relatively low rates of contamination, 10% of the transfusion-associated deaths were due to transfusion-transmitted infections.[12] Bacterial contamination is most common in platelets with a rate of 1 of every 2000 to 3000 transfusions.[30] Between 2011 and 2012, the rate of hepatitis B (HepB) contamination in the US blood supply was estimated to be 0.76 per 10,000 donations; the rate of hepatitis C (HepC), human immunodeficiency virus (HIV), and human T-cell lymphotropic virus (HTLC) was 2.0, 0.28, and 0.34, respectively.[31] Contamination of blood components may arise from an infected donor, introduction of skin flora during donation, improper storage, and contamination from a water bath during the plasma thaw process.[15,24] In the United States, wide-ranging donor screening before donation, systematic testing of the donated blood for infectious diseases, and improved sensitivity of these tests have reduced the risk for transfusion-transmitted infections significantly; the estimated risk for transmission of HepB, HepC, and HIV is estimated at 1:280,000, 1:1,149,000, and 1:1,467,000 donations, respectively.[24]

Transfusion-associated circulatory overload

TACO occurs when the transfused volume produces hydrostatic pulmonary edema; individuals typically develop respiratory distress, hypoxemia, increased central venous pressure, and elevated B-natriuretic peptide concentrations within 2 to 6 hours of transfusion.[15,24] The incidence of TACO is reported to range from 3% to 11%; however, it is likely that TACO is seriously underreported.[32,33] TACO was responsible for 24% of transfusion-related deaths between 2011 and 2015.[12] The risk for TACO increases with recipient age, overall fluid balance, and increase in volume of transfusion, particularly in individuals with comorbid conditions like heart failure, anemia, and chronic pulmonary disease. Diuretics before and during transfusion has been suggested to prevent and effectively manage TACO; furosemide administered intravenously is the drug of choice.[34] Prior prescription of daily diuretic therapy does not prevent TACO however.

Delayed Reactions

Delayed transfusion adverse reactions develop 48 hours or more after transfusion and include erythrocyte and platelet alloimmunization, delayed hemolytic transfusion reactions, posttransfusion purpura, transfusion-related immunomodulation (TRIM), and transfusion-associated graft versus host disease (TA-GVHD; **Table 2**).

Delayed hemolytic transfusion reaction

With erythrocyte and platelet alloimmunization, transfusion recipients have the induction of an immune response, and development of alloantibodies to erythrocytes and/or platelets; this response is triggered by exposure to donor blood cell antigens with

Table 2
Delayed transfusion adverse reactions

Reaction	Signs and Symptoms	Management
Erythrocyte and platelet alloimmunization	Delayed hemolytic transfusion reactions are produced	Decrease alloimmunization by limiting exposure through restrictive transfusion strategies
Delayed hemolytic transfusion reactions	Two to 14 d after transfusion, weakness, jaundice, and elevated bilirubin, anemia, reticulocytosis, spherocytosis, increased lactate dehydrogenase, positive antibody screen, positive DAT	Symptomatic treatment, request antigen-negative components for additional transfusions
Transfusion purpura	Two to 14 d after transfusion, sudden severe thrombocytopenia, petechiae, purpura, mucosal bleeding, diffuse bleeding, platelet-specific antibodies in serum	Typically self-limiting, platelet count recovers within 3 wk, intravenous immunoglobulin with or without corticosteroids, platelet transfusion, without the antigen that produced the reaction
TRIM	Susceptibility to infections, reduced cellular tumor defenses, and enhanced alloimmunization to transfused antigens due to decreased Th1 and Th2 cytokines, impaired delayed-type hypersensitivity skin response, reduced CD8 cells, natural killer cells, CD4 helper T cells, reduced monocyte/macrophage function, decreased cell-mediated cytotoxicity, increased T-regulatory cells and function	Protect individual from exposure to infections while immune compromised
Transfusion-associated graft vs host disease	One to 4 wk after transfusion, pancytopenia, maculopapular rash, vomiting and diarrhea, cholestasis, bone marrow aplasia	Supportive care, no effective treatment, prevent with administration of irradiated components

Data from Dasararaju R, Marques MB. Adverse effects of transfusion. Cancer Control. 2015;22(1):16–25; and American Association of Blood Banks. Circular of information for the use of human blood and blood components. 2016. Available at: https://www.aabb.org/tm/coi/Documents/coi1113.pdf.

transfusion.[35] The titer of these alloantibodies is reduced over time until they are nondetectable. However, subsequent exposure to the antigen causes a secondary immune response in 25 out of 100,000 transfused PRC units, with subsequent hemolysis of erythrocytes and a delayed hemolytic reaction.[36,37] Sensitization to antigens is particularly problematic in those individuals who require chronic transfusions like those with myelodysplastic syndromes and sickle cell anemia. Alloimmunization has been estimated to occur in 3% of individuals who received intensive transfusions (5–20 units in 48 hours) and 15% of patients who received chronic transfusion.[37,38] In patients with sickle cell disease, alloimmunization rates have an incidence of up to

47% depending on patient age, number of red blood cell exposures, and the extent of antigen matching beyond ABO and D.[39]

Posttransfusion purpura

Platelet alloimmunization results in platelet refractoriness as soon as 4 days after transfusion, and potentially life-threatening posttransfusion purpura.[15] Antibody-coated platelets are destroyed by macrophages producing thrombocytopenia; 29% of individuals receiving chronic transfusions who were refractory to platelet transfusion were found to have significant levels of antiplatelet antibodies.[40] Platelet refractoriness is diagnosed when individual response (10 minutes to 1 hour) to 2 sequential platelet transfusions is inadequate ($<5 \times 10^9$/L).[41] Posttransfusion purpura occurs about a week after transfusion and is due to severe thrombocytopenia secondary to immune platelet destruction; the incidence of this reaction is approximately 1 in 50,000 to 100,000 transfusions and multiparous women are more likely to be affected.[42]

Transfusion-related immunomodulation

TRIM is an immune suppression that occurs after transfusion of blood. In fact, blood transfusion was previously used as an immune suppressant for early renal transplant patients to improve immediate graft survival.[43] Evidence demonstrated that TRIM is associated with transfusion of allogeneic leukocytes; the resultant immune suppression is due in part to suppression of cytotoxic cells and monocyte activity, increased release of prostaglandins, alteration in concentrations of proinflammatory and anti-inflammatory cytokines and eicosanoids, and increased suppressor T-cell activity.[44] The consequences include greater susceptibility to infection, reduced cellular tumor defenses, and enhanced alloimmunization to transfused antigens.[45]

Transfusion-associated graft versus host disease

TA-GVHD occurs in immune-compromised and some immune-competent individuals who receive a transfusion with viable recipient T lymphocytes; these donor lymphocytes replicate and mount an immune response against recipient cells. Because of the inability of the recipient to fight this immune response, the donor cells essentially attack the recipient tissues.[46,47] TA-GVHD can occur at any point between 2 days and 6 weeks after transfusion and produces fever, rash, hepatomegaly with liver dysfunction, pancytopenia, and the presence of leukocyte chimerism. There is no effective treatment, and mortality approaches 90%; thus, prevention is vital. Gamma and UV radiation of blood components have been used to prevent TA-GVHD.

BEST PRACTICES TO PREVENT OR MANAGE ADVERSE REACTIONS TO TRANSFUSION
Leukoreduction and Irradiation Before Transfusion

Donor leukocytes in transfused components are associated with multiple adverse reactions; these include FNHTR, TA-GVHD, alloimmunization, and transmission of cytomegalovirus in at-risk patients.[45] Leukoreduction, removal of 99.9% of leukocytes through filtration, may prevent these events and subsequent worse outcomes.[45,48] Leukoreduction can be performed within 24 hours of donation, prestorage leukoreduction, or pretransfusion at the bedside. Quality guidelines for leukoreduction indicate the maximum number of leukocytes that should remain in whole blood, PRCs, pooled platelets, and plasma after leukoreduction are less than 5×10^6/L[49,50]; however, the leukocyte threshold for development of TA-GVHD is not known.[51] Previously, scientists reported benefits of leukoreduction from primarily retrospective and observational studies; after universal leukoreduction, decreased prevalence in TRALI up to 83%, in TACO up to 49%, and a 35% reduction in febrile FNTR were reported,[52] and mortality was decreased by 13%.[53] However, in a recent *Cochrane Review* that included 13 studies, Simancas-Racines and colleagues[54] concluded that leukoreduction produced no patient harm, but there was no evidence to support benefit either. Outcomes evaluated included multiple adverse effects including TRALI and TACO, infectious and non-infectious complications, and mortality. Evaluation of study quality determined that investigations were very low to low quality; thus, well-designed, prospective studies are needed to truly evaluate efficacy.

The exposure of blood components to gamma UV radiation before transfusion prevents the development of TA-GVHD. Exposure of PRCs and platelets to radiation damages lymphocyte DNA and prevents mitotic activity after transfusion.[55] Irradiated components should be administered to all individuals at high risk for TA-GVHD (**Box 1**). Irradiation reduces the storage life of PRCs from 42 to 28 days, may decrease erythrocyte efficacy after transfusion by about 25%, increases the amount of free hemoglobin, and significantly enhances potassium leak from erythrocytes.[56] Although originally thought that irradiation had no negative effects on platelets, Julmy and colleagues[51] found that platelets irradiated the day of transfusion had a 7% higher efficacy after transfusion compared with those irradiated before the day of transfusion.

Storage Age of Blood Products Before Transfusion

PRCs and platelets undergo cellular alterations that begin at time of storage and worsen linearly with increased storage time.[57,58] Major changes associated with this storage lesion include depletion of adenosine triphosphate, breakdown of the cell Na^+/K^+ pump, a change in cell membrane structure and overall shape from a smooth, flexible structure to a round, hardened structure with protrusions, breakdown of the

---

Box 1
Indications for administration of irradiated blood components

Blood component to be transfused donated by family member

Blood component from HLA-selected donor

Blood component from directed donor with possible familial relationship

Intrauterine transfusion

Exchange transfusion in neonates

Congenital immune deficiency

Acute leukemia: HLA matched or family donated components

Hodgkin disease

Treatment with purine analogues and related medications (fludarabine, 2CDA, deoxycoformycin, clofarabine, bendamustine, nelarabine)

Treatment with atemtuzumab

Immunocompromised stem cell recipients

Organ transplant recipients

Individuals who require bone marrow transplantation in near future

Individuals with thymic hypoplasia, Wiskott-Aldrich syndrome, Leiner disease, 5'nucleotidase deficiency

Chronic lymphocytic leukemia

Data from Carson JL, Grossman BJ, Kleinman S, et al. Red blood cell transfusion: a clinical practice guideline from the AABB*. Ann Intern Med 2012;157(1):49–58.

cell membrane and subsequent cellular swelling with release of intracellular contents, increase in extracellular potassium and subsequent decrease in pH of the unit, and depletion of 2,3-diphosphoglycerate, a metabolic byproduct that alters hemoglobin release of oxygen to cells.[57,58] The clinical consequences of the storage lesion may include significant loss of erythrocytes after transfusion, reduction in microcirculatory flow, coagulopathy, endothelial dysfunction, immune suppression, cellular hypoxia, and systemic inflammation.[59] However, investigators of a recent systematic review and meta-analysis of 12 randomized trials with more than 5200 patients across multiple clinical populations concluded there was no effect of age of transfused components on patient mortality (relative risk [RR] 1.04, 95% confidence interval [CI] 0.94–1.14, $P = .45$) or adverse events (RR 1.02, 95% CI 0.91–1.14, $P = .74$).[60] The 2016 clinical practice guidelines from the American Association of Blood Banks (AABB) stated that the current evidence to support the benefit of newer PRCs over older units was insufficient.[61,62]

There is limited evidence about the platelet storage lesion, but issues related to storage of platelets are also more complicated; platelets must be stored at room temperature, which increases the risk for bacterial growth.[63] Platelet activation capacity was shown to be significantly higher on day 0 compared with day 3 of storage (39.87% ± 11.47% vs 2.43% ± 0.79%, $P<.05$), and phosphatidylserine, a marker of cell apoptosis, was 6-fold higher by day 3 as compared with day 0 (1.36% vs 6.15%, $P<.05$).[64] This biomarker peaked by day 7 of storage (9.83%), demonstrating greater cell death with longer storage. However, investigators have identified no difference in patient mortality based on the age of platelets transfused for critically injured trauma patients. These investigators did identify a higher rate of overall complications in patients who received platelets stored for 5 days (29.2%) compared with platelets stored for 4 days (19.3%) or ≤3 days (13.3%, $P = .005$).[65] Current clinical practice guidelines do not address storage age of platelets.[63] Thus, additional evidence for the impact of the storage lesion on adverse outcomes in critically ill patients is needed. Current guidelines identify the appropriate storage time and temperature for blood components (**Table 3**).

Premedication Before Transfusion

In the United States, an estimated 50% of in-hospital transfusions are preceded by premedication with an antipyretic and antihistamine to reduce the likelihood of allergic and FNHTRs.[67] However, research evidence to date does not support this intervention. A *Cochrane Review* of 3 randomized controlled trials found that premedication with acetaminophen and diphenhydramine did not reduce the risk of allergic reactions or FNHTRs compared with placebo[68]; there was no statistically significant difference in allergic reactions (RR 0.13, 95% CI 0.01–2.39, RR 1.46, 95% CI 0.78–2.73) and febrile reactions (RR 0.52, 95% CI 0.22–1.26) with premedication. There was a significant difference in the likelihood of a febrile transfusion reaction when diphenhydramine was compared with hydrocortisone premedication (odds ratio [OR] 2.38, 95% CI 1.07–5.27). A recent systematic review[69] also concluded that premedication with acetaminophen and diphenhydramine was not supported as a strategy to reduce reactions when leukoreduction was universal. Thus, premedication with these drugs is not recommended.

Pretransfusion administration of furosemide is intended to reduce TACO. The hypothesized rationale for premedication with a loop diuretic is based primarily on the action of the drug to block the Na-K-Cl$_2$ cotransporter in the thick ascending loop of Henle, which increases water excretion and subsequent extracellular and pulmonary interstitial fluid volume; furosemide also produces shifts in alveolar fluid to the intravascular space, produces venodilation, and improves lung compliance. Recently, Lieberman and colleagues[33] retrospectively evaluated TACO cases and found that age older than 70 years, renal dysfunction, and history of heart failure were common risk factors; the median volume of blood prescribed and crystalloid/colloid infused in the preceding 24 hours was 500 mL and 2200 mL, respectively. Furosemide 20 mg was prescribed in 29% of cases and administered typically halfway through or upon completion the transfusion. These investigators concluded that inadequate premedication with furosemide may have contributed to the development of TACO. However, in a recent *Cochrane Review*, Sarai and Tejani[70] evaluated data from 4 small trials and concluded that there was inadequate evidence to support the standard use of furosemide to prevent TACO. These trials were small and underpowered, and TACO was not a primary outcome. Thus, high-quality trials are needed to determine whether furosemide is effective in the prevention of TACO, and if so, the appropriate dose and timing of administration in relation to transfusion.

Restrictive Transfusion Practices

In 1942, Adams and Lundy[71] proposed the 10/30 clinical standard for transfusion of blood components; when hemoglobin concentration was $\leq$10 g/dL or hematocrit less than 30%, patients required transfusion. However, blood components are a resource dependent on donation from primarily altruistic individuals in developed countries; in underdeveloped countries, donation and storage ability may be scarce. Additional concerns about adverse reactions and costs led to evaluation of transfusion practice. In 1988, the National Institutes of Health Consensus Conference concluded that the use of one criterion for transfusion need was not warranted.[72] In 2004, the CRIT studies performed with data from 213 US hospitals found that mean hemoglobin trigger for transfusion was 8.6 $\pm$ 1.7 g/dL.[73] Several clinical trials ensued that tested a liberal transfusion trigger of 10 g/dL with a restrictive trigger, usually 7 or 8 g/dL. Investigators for the Transfusion Requirements after Cardiac Surgery trial found no difference in 30-day mortality (5%, 95% CI 2%–7% vs 6%, 95% CI, 3%–9%, P = .93), cardiogenic shock (5%, 95% CI 2%–7% vs 9%, 95% CI, 5%–12%, P = .42), ARDS (1%, 95% CI, 0%–2% vs 2%, 95% CI, 0%–4%, P = .99), or acute renal failure requiring dialysis or hemofiltration (5%, 95% CI 2%–9% vs 4%, 95% CI 2%–6%, P = .99) in cardiac surgery patients.[74] However, transfusion of 5 or more units of PRCs was associated with a 25% increase in mortality (OR 1.25, 95% CI 1.09–1.42, P = .001). In a multicenter trial, investigators found no difference in long-term mortality (median 3.1 years follow up) (HR 1.09, 95% CI 0·95–1·25, P = 0.21) in high-risk patients 50 years of age and older after surgery to repair a hip fracture.[75] Recently, investigators for a 2016 *Cochrane Review* evaluated data from 31 high-quality trials with 12,587 participants from a wide range of specialties that tested a liberal versus restrictive transfusion strategy (trigger hemoglobin 7–8 g/dL); these investigators found that restrictive transfusion strategies reduced the likelihood of transfusion by 43% (RR 0.57, 95% CI 0.49–0.65) and did not influence 30-day mortality, rates of cardiovascular complications, thromboembolism, and pneumonia. Thus, the evidence to support a restrictive transfusion strategy in these populations is well supported with evidence (see **Table 3**).

Donor and Blood Screening Procedures

To ensure that blood components are safe for transfusion, The FDA and AABB established criteria for donation and testing of donated blood before transfusion[50]; these criteria are updated as new knowledge about transmission of disease is developed. Donor criteria address age (16 or older but may differ by state), self-report of good health on day of donation, recent health and medication history, history of prior

Table 3
Guidelines for blood component transfusion

Blood Product	Storage Time	Transfusion	
		Do	**Do not**
Packed red blood cells[61]	Stored at 1–6°C for 35–42 d depending on preservation solution	Adhere to a restrictive transfusion threshold (7 g/dL) for *hospitalized adult patients who are hemodynamically stable*, including critically ill patients (evidence: moderate; strong recommendation)[a] Adhere to a transfusion threshold of 8 g/dL for *patients undergoing orthopedic or cardiac surgery and those with preexisting cardiovascular disease* (evidence: moderate; strong recommendation)[a] Use any PRBC unit within the specified licensed date before expiration (evidence: moderate; strong recommendation)	Preferentially choose PRBC units based on length of storage (ie, <10 d), exception may be neonates Transfuse when the anemia may be corrected with iron, B$_{12}$, folate, and so forth Transfuse because a patient is hypotensive in the absence of symptomatic anemia
FFP[66]	May be frozen for up to 1 y; should be transfused immediately; must be discarded within 24 h of thawing (may have variance that allows use up to 5 d after thaw)	Transfuse trauma patients requiring massive transfusion (evidence: moderate) Transfuse patients with warfarin anticoagulation-related intracranial hemorrhage (evidence: low)	No recommendations for or against transfusion of FFP at an FFP:PRBC ratio of 1:3 or more in trauma patients during massive transfusion (evidence: low) No recommendations for or against FFP transfusion in patients undergoing surgery in the absence of massive transfusion (evidence: low) No recommendations for or against FFP transfusion to reverse warfarin in patients without intracranial hemorrhage (evidence: very low) Do not transfuse FFP in other groups where data were available (acute pancreatitis, organophosphate poisoning, coagulopathy associated with acetaminophen overdose, intracranial hemorrhage after severe closed head injury in patients without coagulopathy, nonsurgical noncardiac patients in the intensive care unit; evidence: very low)

| Platelets[63] | Stored at room temperature for a maximum of 5 d | Prophylactically transfuse hospitalized adult patients with a platelet count of ≤10 × 10^9 cells/L to reduce the risk of spontaneous bleeding with up to a single apheresis unit or equivalent (evidence: moderate; strong recommendation) Prophylactically transfuse patients having elective central venous catheter placement with a platelet count of <20 × 10^9 cells/L (evidence: low; weak recommendation) Prophylactically transfuse patients having elective diagnostic lumbar puncture with a platelet count of <50 × 10^9 cells/L (evidence: very low; weak recommendation) Prophylactically transfuse patients having major elective nonneuraxial surgery with a platelet count <50 × 10^9 cells/L (evidence: very low; weak recommendation) Transfuse patients having cardiopulmonary bypass who exhibit perioperative bleeding with thrombocytopenia and/or with evidence of platelet dysfunction (evidence: very low; weak recommendation) | Prophylactically transfuse patients who are nonthrombocytopenic and have cardiac surgery with cardiopulmonary bypass (evidence: very low; weak recommendation) No recommendations for patients receiving antiplatelet therapy who have intracranial hemorrhage (traumatic or spontaneous; evidence: very low; uncertain recommendation) |

Abbreviation: PRBCs, packed red blood cells.
a Applicable to all but the following conditions, for which evidence is insufficient to provide recommendations: acute coronary syndrome, severe thrombocytopenia, and chronic transfusion-dependent anemia.

donations, and potential exposures to blood-borne pathogens that include bacterial, viral, protozoa, and prion disorders. Every unit of donated blood is systematically tested to determine the ABO blood group, Rh type, presence of atypical erythrocyte antibodies, and for bacteria, viruses and protozoa (**Box 2**). Tests are added and analysis techniques updated as evidence of transmission via blood is supported and test sensitivity is improved.[76] Investigators have identified reductions in rates of hepB and hepC in donated blood in the United States, but increased rates of HIV and HTLV; however, rates for HIV, HepC, and HTLV in donor blood are less than 1 per million donations.[77] Despite the improved safety of donated blood, the US population continues to perceive high risk with blood transfusion, except when autologous blood is used.[78]

Cell Salvage or Autotransfusion

Cell salvage is the collection of autologous blood lost during surgery or after trauma, with subsequent autotransfusion to the patient. Cell savage is intended to reduce the use of donor blood and minimize adverse reactions to allogeneic transfusion.[79] Prior investigators estimated that cell salvage and autotransfusion reduced the use of allogeneic blood use by 6500 to 320,000 units per year.[80] Recently, Rasouli and colleagues[81] found that autologous blood transfusion reduced the need for allogeneic transfusion by 16% (OR 0.84, 95% CI 0.82–0.85, $P<.001$) after joint arthroplasty. Results from the most recent *Cochrane Review* of cell salvage and autotransfusion included 75 trials conducted in patients during orthopedic and cardiac surgery. Investigators demonstrated that allogeneic transfusions were reduced by 38% (RR 0.62: 95% CI 0.55–0.70); the use of allogeneic blood was reduced by 0.68 units per patient, and autologous transfusion did not affect clinical outcomes. However, the quality of these trials was poor with high risk of bias.[82] Unfortunately, only one very small study (n = 44) focused on the use of cell salvage and autotransfusion in the trauma population[83]; investigators found no difference in mortality (OR 1.07, 95% CI 0.31–3.72), adverse events (OR 0.54, 95% CI 0.11–2.55), and costs. An average of 4.7 units of allogeneic transfusion was required for those in the cell salvage group compared with control. Thus, evidence for cell salvage and autotransfusion require high-quality clinical trials in diverse populations to support their efficacy.

Box 2
Infectious diseases for donor blood screening
HepB
HepC
HIV
HTLV-1, -2
Treponema pallidum (syphilis)
Trypanosoma cruzi
West Nile virus
Cytomegalovirus
Zika virus
From U.S. Food and Drug Administration. Complete List of Donor Screening Assays for Infectious Agents and HIV Diagnostic Assays. 2016. Available at: http://www.fda.gov/biologicsbloodvaccines/bloodbloodproducts/approvedproducts/licensedproductsblas/blooddonorscreening/infectiousdisease/ucm080466.htm; with permission.

Reduction of Iatrogenic Anemia

Iatrogenic anemia is attributed to frequent phlebotomy and removal of blood for diagnostic testing. Salisbury and colleagues[84] found that for each 50 mL of blood removed from patients after acute myocardial infarction, the risk of moderate to severe iatrogenic anemia increased by 18%. Another analysis by this group[85] found that moderate and severe iatrogenic anemia increased the likelihood of in-hospital mortality by 38% and 339%, respectively (moderate OR 1.38, 95% CI 1.10–1.73, severe OR 3.39, 95% CI 2.59–4.44) compared with those with no anemia. Investigators for a review of 9 studies of phlebotomy conservation strategies concluded that reduction in number of ordered laboratory tests, the use of blood conservation devices for diagnostic sampling, and education about iatrogenic anemia and its consequences should be used to improve practice and patient outcomes.[86] Currently, there is a lack of evidence to demonstrate efficacy of blood conservation devices, education about iatrogenic anemia and associated outcomes, and the impact of standards for decreased blood volume for diagnostic testing in the critical care unit.

SUMMARY

Transfusion of blood components is associated with several adverse reactions, both acute and delayed, that may be mild to life-threatening. There are several strategies and guidelines in place that intend to reduce the need for, and the safety of, transfused blood components; however, not all are supported by rigorous research. Although the evidence to support restrictive transfusion approaches is from high-quality trials, rigorous clinical trials are still needed to evaluate the efficacy of many of these strategies.

REFERENCES

1. American Red Cross. Blood facts and statistics. 2016. Available at: http://www.redcrossblood.org/learn-about-blood/blood-facts-and-statistics.   Accessed November 19, 2016.
2. Lelubre C, Vincent JL. Red blood cell transfusion in the critically ill patient. Ann Intensive Care 2011;1:43.
3. Hayden SJ, Albert TJ, Watkins TR, et al. Anemia in critical illness; insights into etiology, consequences, and management. Am J Respir Crit Care Med 2012; 185(10):1049–57.
4. Jakacka N, Snarski E, Mekuria S. Prevention of iatrogenic anemia in critical and neonatal care. Adv Clin Exp Med 2016;25:191–7.
5. Politis C, Wiersum JC, Richardson C, et al. The International Haemovigilane Network Database for the surveillance of adverse reactions and events in donors and recipients of blood components: technical issues and results. Vox Sang 2016;111:409–17.
6. Harvey AR, Basavaraju SV, Chung KW, et al. Transfusion-related adverse reactions reported to the National Healthcare Safety Network Hemovigilance Module, United States, 2010 to 2012. Transfusion 2015;55(4):709–18.
7. Learoyd P. The history of blood transfusion prior to the 20th century–part 1. Transfus Med 2012;22(5):308–14.
8. Learoyd P. The history of blood transfusion prior to the 20th century–part 2. Transfus Med 2012;22(6):372–6.
9. Giangrande PL. The history of blood transfusion. Br J Haematol 2000;110(4): 758–67.

10. Farr AD. Blood group serology—the first four decades (1900-1939). Med Hist 1979;23(2):215–26.
11. Alter HJ, Klein HG. The hazards of blood transfusion in historical perspective. Blood 2008;112(7):2617–26.
12. U.S. Food and Drug Administration. Fatalities Reported to FDA Following Blood Collection and Transfusion Annual Summary for FY 2015. 2016. Available at: http://www.fda.gov/downloads/BiologicsBloodVaccines/SafetyAvailability/ReportaProblem/TransfusionDonationFatalities/UCM518148.pdf. Accessed October 18, 2016.
13. Kumar R, Gupta M, Gupta V, et al. Acute transfusion reactions (ATRs) in intensive care unit (ICU): a retrospective study. J Clin Diagn Res 2014;8(2):127–9.
14. Badami KG, Joliffe E, Stephens M. Transfusion-associated dyspnea–shadow or substance? Vox Sang 2015;109(2):197–200.
15. Dasararaju R, Marques MB. Adverse effects of transfusion. Cancer Control 2015; 22(1):16–25.
16. Strobel E. Hemolytic transfusion reactions. Transfus Med Hemother 2008;35: 346–53.
17. Flegel WA. Pathogenesis and mechanism of antibody-mediated hemolysis. Transfusion 2015;55(Suppl):S47–58.
18. Sovic D, Dodig J, Banovic M, et al. Transfusion treatment at Sestre Milosrdnice University Hospital Center during a twelve-year period. Acta Clin Croat 2015; 53(3):342–7.
19. Rajesh K, Harsh S, Amarjit K. Effects of prestorage leukoreduction on the rate of febrile nonhemolytic transfusion reactions to red blood cells in a tertiary care hospital. Ann Med Health Sci Res 2015;5(3):185–8.
20. Menitove JE, McElligott MC, Aster RH. Febrile transfusion reaction: what component should be given next? Vox Sang 1982;42:318–21.
21. King KE, Shirey RS, Thoman SK, et al. Universal leukoreduction decreases the incidence of febrile nonhemolytic transfusion reactions to RBCs. Transfusion 2004;44(1):25–9.
22. McFaul SJ, Corley JB, Mester CW, et al. Packed blood cells stored in AS-5 become proinflammatory during storage. Transfusion 2009;49(7):1451–60.
23. Menis M, Forshee RA, Anderson SA, et al. Febrile non-haemolytic transfusion reaction occurrence and potential risk factors among the U.S. elderly transfused in the inpatient setting, as recorded in Medicare databases during 2011-2012. Vox Sang 2015;108(3):251–61.
24. Pandey S, Vyas GN. Adverse effects of plasma transfusion. Transfusion 2012; 53(suppl 1):65S–79S.
25. van Tilborogh-de Jong AJ, Wiersum-Osselton JC, Touw DJ, et al. Presence of medication taken by donors in plasma for transfusion. Vox Sang 2015;108(4): 323–7.
26. Hirayama F. Current understanding of allergic transfusion reactions: incidence, pathogenesis, laboratory tests, prevention and treatment. Br J Haematol 2013; 160:434–44.
27. Cohn CS, Stubbs J, Schwartz J, et al. A comparison of adverse reaction rates for PAS C versus plasma platelet units. Transfusion 2014;54(8):1927–34.
28. Clifford I, Jia Q, Subramanian A, et al. Characterizing the epidemiology of postoperative transfusion-related acute lung injury. Transfusion 2015a;122(1):12–20.
29. Storch EK, Hillyer CD, Shaz BH. Spotlight on pathogenesis of TRALI: HNA-3a (CTL2) antibodies. Blood 2014;124(12):1868–72.

30. Centers for Disease Control and Prevention. Blood safety. 2016. Available at: http://www.cdc.gov/bloodsafety/bbp/diseases_organisms.html. Accessed November 19, 2016.
31. Dodd RY, Notari EP, Nelson D, et al. Development of a multisystem surveillance database for transfusion-transmitted infections among blood donors in the United States. Transfusion 2016;56:2781–9.
32. Clifford L, Qing J, Hemang Y, et al. Characterizing the epidemiology of perioperative transfusion-associated circulatory overload. Anesthesiology 2015;122(1): 21–8.
33. Lieberman L, Maskens C, Cserti-Gazdewich C, et al. A retrospective review of patient factors, transfusion practices, and outcomes in patients with transfusion-associated circulatory overload. Transfus Med Rev 2013;27(4): 206–12.
34. Alam A, Lin Y, Lima A, et al. The prevention of transfusion-associated circulatory overload. Transfus Med Rev 2013;27(2):105–12.
35. Zimring JC, Weniak L, Semple JW, et al. Current problems and future directions of transfusion-induced alloimmunization: summary of an NHLBI working group. Transfusion 2011;52(2):435–41.
36. Rogers MA, Rohde JM, Blumberg N. Haemovigilance of reactions associated with red blood cell transfusion: comparison across 17 countries. Vox Sang 2016;110(3):266–77.
37. Sanz C, Nomdedeu M, Belkaid M, et al. Red blood cell alloimmunization in transfused patients with myelodysplastic syndrome or chronic myelomonocytic leukemia. Transfusion 2013;53(4):710–5.
38. Zalpuri S, Middelburg RA, Schonewille H, et al. Intensive red blood cell transfusions and risk of alloimmunization. Transfusion 2014;54(2):278–84.
39. Chou ST, Jackson T, Vege S, et al. High prevalence of red blood cell alloimmunization in sickle cell disease despite transfusion from Rh-matched minority donors. Blood 2013;122(6):1062–71.
40. Jia Y, Li W, Liu N, et al. Prevalence of platelet-specific antibodies and efficacy of crossmatch-compatible platelet transfusions in refractory patients. Transfus Med 2014;24(6):406–10.
41. Forest SK, Hod EA. Management of the platelet refractory patient. Hematol Oncol Clin North Am 2016;30(3):665–77.
42. Padhi P, Parihar GS, Stepp J, et al. Post-transfusion purpura: a rare and life-threatening aetiology of thrombocytopenia. BMJ Case Rep 2013;2013 [pii: bcr2013008860].
43. Refaai MA, Blumberg N. Transfusion immunomodulation from a clinical perspective: an update. Expert Rev Hematol 2013;6(6):653–63.
44. Cata JP, Wang H, Gottumukkala V, et al. Inflammatory response, immunosuppression, and cancer recurrence after perioperative blood transfusion. Anaesthesia 2013;110(5):690–701.
45. Lannan K, Sahler J, Spinelli SL, et al. Transfusion immunomodulation–the case for leukoreduced and (perhaps) washed transfusions. Blood Cells Mol Dis 2013; 50(1):61–8.
46. Kopolovic I, Ostro J, Tsubota H, et al. A systematic review of transfusion-associated graft-versus-host disease. Blood 2015;126:406–14.
47. Prichard AE, Shaz BH. Survey of irradiation practice for the prevention of transfusion-associated graft-versus-host disease. Arch Pathol Lab Med 2016; 140(10):1092–7.

48. U.S. Food and Drug Administration. Guidance for industry: pre-storage leukocyte reduction of whole blood and blood components intended for transfusion. 2016. Available at: http://www.fda.gov/BiologicsBloodVaccines/GuidanceCompliance RegulatoryInformation/Guidances/Blood/ucm320636.htm. Accessed November 19, 2016.

49. American Association of Blood Banks . Circular of information for the use of human blood and blood components. 2016. Available at: https://www.aabb.org/tm/coi/Documents/coi1113.pdf. Accessed October 18, 2016.

50. American Association of Blood Banks. Blood donor screening and testing. 2016b. Available at: http://www.aabb.org/advocacy/regulatorygovernment/donoreligibility/Pages/default.aspx. Accessed October 18, 2016.

51. Julmy F, Ammann RA, Fontana S, et al. Transfusion efficacy of apheresis platelet concentrates irradiated at the day of transfusion is superior compared to platelets irradiated in advance. Transfus Med Hemother 2014;41:176–81.

52. Blumberg N, Heal JM, Gettings KF, et al. An association between decreased cardiopulmonary complications (transfusion-related acute lung injury and transfusion-associated circulatory overload) and implementation of universal leukoreduction of blood transfusions. Transfusion 2010;50(12):2738–44.

53. Hebert PC, Fergusson D, Blajchman MA, et al. Clinical outcomes following institution of the Canadian universal leukoreduction program for red blood cell transfusions. JAMA 2003;289(15):1941–9.

54. Simancas-Racines D, Osorio D, Marti-Carvajal AJ, et al. Leukoreduction for the prevention of adverse reactions from allogeneic blood transfusion. Cochrane Database Syst Rev 2015;(12):CD009745.

55. Moroff G, Luban NLC. The irradiation of blood and blood components to prevent graft-versus-host disease: technical issues and guidelines. Transfus Med Rev 1997;11(1):15–26.

56. Treleaven J, Gennery A, Marsh J, et al. Guidelines on the use of irradiated blood components prepared by the British Committee for Standards in Haematology blood transfusion task force. Br J Haematol 2010;152:35–51.

57. Orlov D, Karkouti K. The pathophysiology and consequences of red blood cell storage. Anaesthesia 2015;70(Suppl 1):e9–12.

58. Shrivastava M. The platelet storage lesion. Transfus Apheresis Sci 2009;41(2):105–13.

59. Qu L, Triulzi DJ. Clinical effects of red blood cell storage. Cancer Control 2015;22(1):26–37.

60. Alexander PE, Barty R, Fei Y, et al. Transfusion of fresher vs older red blood cells in hospitalized patients: a systematic review and meta-analysis. Blood 2016;127(4):400–10.

61. Carson JL, Stanworth SJ, Roubinian N, et al. Transfusion thresholds and other strategies for guiding allogeneic red blood cell transfusion. Cochrane Database Syst Rev 2016;(10):CD002042.

62. Carless PA, Henry DA, Carson JL, et al. Transfusion thresholds and other strategies for guiding allogeneic red blood cell transfusion. Cochrane Database Syst Rev 2010;(10):CD002042.

63. Kaufman RM, Djulbegovic B, Gernsheimer T, et al. Platelet transfusion: a clinical practice guideline from the AABB. Ann Intern Med 2015;162(3):205–13.

64. Perales Villarroel JP, Figueredo R, Guan Y, et al. Increased platelet storage time is associated with mitochondrial dysfunction and impaired platelet function. J Surg Res 2013;184(1):422–9.

65. Inaba K, Branco BC, Rhee P, et al. Impact of the duration of platelet storage in critically ill trauma patients. J Trauma 2011;71(6):1766–73 [discussion: 1773–4].
66. Roback JD, Caldwell S, Carson J, et al. Evidence-based practice guidelines for plasma transfusion. Transfusion 2010;50(6):1227–39.
67. Geiger TL, Howard SC. Acetaminophen and diphenhydramine premedication for allergic and febrile nonhemolytic transfusion reactions: good prophylaxis or bad practice? Transfus Med Rev 2007;21:1–12.
68. Marti-Carvajal AJ, Sola I, Gonzalez LE, et al. Pharmacological interventions for the prevention of allergic and febrile non-haemolytic transfusion reactions. Cochrane Database Syst Rev 2010;(6):CD007539.
69. Duran J, Siddique S, Cleary M. Effects of leukoreduction and premedication with acetaminophen and diphenhydramine in minimizing febrile nonhemolytic transfusion reactions and allergic transfusion reactions during and after blood product administration: a literature review with recommendations for practice. J Pediatr Oncol Nurs 2014;31(4):223–9.
70. Sarai M, Tejani AM. Loop diuretics for patients receiving blood transfusions. Cochrane Database Syst Rev 2015;(2):CD010138.
71. Adams RC, Lundy JS. Anesthesia in cases of poor surgical risk. Some suggestions for decreasing the risk. Surg Gynecol Obstet 1942;74:1011–9.
72. Perioperative red cell transfusion. Natl Inst Health Consens Dev Conf Consens Statement 1988;7(4):1–19. Available at: https://consensus.nih.gov/1988/1988redcelltransfusion070html.htm.
73. Corwin HL, Gettinger A, Pearl RG, et al. The CRIT study: anemia and blood transfusion in the critically ill—current clinical practice in the United States. Crit Care Med 2004;32(1):39–52.
74. Hajjar LA, Vincent JL, Galas FR, et al. Transfusion requirements after cardiac surgery: the TRACS randomized controlled trial. J Am Med Assoc 2010;304(14):1559–67.
75. Carson JL, Sieber F, Cook DR, et al. Liberal versus restrictive blood transfusion strategy: 3-year survival and cause of death results from the FOCUS randomized controlled trial. Lancet 2015;385(9974):1183–9.
76. American Red Cross. Blood testing. 2016. Available at: http://www.redcrossblood.org/learn-about-blood/what-happens-donated-blood/blood-testing. Accessed November 19, 2016.
77. Zou S, Stamer SL, Dodd RY. Donor testing and risk: current prevalence, incidence, and residual risk of transfusion-transmissible agents in US allogeneic donations. Transfus Med Rev 2012;26(2):119–28.
78. Ngo LT, Bruhn R, Custer B. Risk perception and its role in attitudes toward blood transfusion: a qualitative systematic review. Transfus Med Rev 2013;27(2):119–28.
79. Schoettker P, Marcucci CE, Casso G, et al. Revisiting transfusion safety and alternatives to transfusion. La Presse Medicale 2016;45(7–8 Pt 2):e331–40.
80. Davies L, Brown TJ, Haynes S, et al. Cost-effectiveness of cell salvage and alternative methods of minimising perioperative allogeneic blood transfusion: a systematic review and economic model. Health Technol Assess 2006;10(44):1–228.
81. Rasouli MR, Maltenfort MG, Erkocak OF, et al. Blood management after total joint arthroplasty in the United States: 19-year trend analysis. Transfusion 2016;56(5):1112–20.
82. Carless PA, Henry DA, Moxey AJ, et al. Cell salvage for minimising perioperative allogeneic blood transfusion. Cochrane Database Syst Rev 2010;(4):CD001888.

83. Li J, Sun SL, Tian JH, et al. Cell salvage in emergency trauma surgery. Cochrane Database Syst Rev 2015;(1):CD007379.

84. Salisbury AC, Reid KJ, Alexander KP, et al. Diagnostic blood loss from phlebotomy and hospital-acquired anemia during acute myocardial infarction. Arch Intern Med 2011;171(18):1646–53.

85. Salisbury AC, Reid KJ, Alexander KP, et al. Hospital-acquired anemia and in-hospital mortality in patients with acute myocardial infarction. Am Heart J 2011; 162:300–9.

86. Page C, Retter A, Wyncoll D. Blood conservation devices in critical care: a narrative review. Ann Intensive Care 2013;3:14.

Alternative to Blood Replacement in the Critically Ill

Deborah J. Tolich, DNP, RN*, Kelly McCoy, BSN, RN

KEYWORDS

- Blood transfusion • Blood management • Blood alternatives
- Transfusion alternatives

KEY POINTS

- Blood volumes can be managed with a patient-specific approach.
- Blood transfusion and anemia are common in critical illness.
- Iatrogenic blood loss can be reduced.
- Progress has been made in manufactured blood products.
- Prevention and critical anemia protocol are followed when blood is not an option.

INTRODUCTION

Anemia and the need for blood transfusions in critical illness is a common occurrence.[1] Patients become anemic through multiple causative factors: blood loss, increased phlebotomy, decreased red blood cell (RBC) production, and longevity. Blood transfusions have been associated with poorer outcomes, warranting the inclusion of non-blood therapies and strategies in managing patient blood volume. A conference on transfusion outcomes reported 88% of blood transfusions were associated with a worse outcome or provided no benefit.[2] The *Circular of Information for the Use of Human Blood and Blood Components* (2016) reports the indication for RBC transfusion is a critical or symptomatic insufficiency of oxygen-carrying capacity and red cell exchange transfusion.[3] RBC transfusions are not indicated for anemia that can be treated with hematinic medications or as primary treatment of volume expansion and a mechanism to increase oncotic pressure.

The American Board of Internal Medicine Foundation initiated the Choosing Wisely campaign to lower the overutilization of testing and procedures. Within the campaign,

Disclosure Statement: No disclosures.
Blood Management, Cleveland Clinic Health System, 9500 Euclid Avenue, Cleveland, OH 44195, USA
* Corresponding author.
E-mail address: detoli@ccf.org

ccnursing.theclinics.com

blood transfusion as the most performed procedure in the United States included the following[4]:

- Dosing of blood products
- Correction of nutritional deficiencies in stable patients instead of transfusion
- Advisement against the use of blood products to reverse warfarin
- Elimination of serial blood testing in stable patients
- Refrain from transfusing O blood to non-O except in emergencies for women of childbearing age without blood group identification.

Nonblood treatments or strategies are centralized in minimizing blood loss, restoration and maintenance of intravascular volume, and accelerating production of RBCs. Situations may arise in which blood transfusion is not an option, such as patients having multiple alloantibodies so that it becomes difficult to obtain cross-matched blood products, or patients may decline the use of blood products due to personal or religious belief. Patient blood management (PBM) uses multiple modalities to achieve the best patient outcomes for all patients regardless of ability to receive blood transfusions. There are several tenets within blood management (**Box 1**). The primary pillars are described as anemia tolerance, management of bleeding, and supporting erythropoiesis.[5] The art of medical practice is in the selection of the right combination of therapies. This is complex due to the number of potential patient variables and is open to wide differences in practice. Therefore, several items should be taken into consideration when contemplating a cellular or acellular transplant of blood products and a PBM plan of care (**Box 2**).

IATROGENIC ANEMIA

Iatrogenic anemia can be defined as anemia caused by hospital procedures, not by patient illness. A recent article reported that 74% of patients admitted to the hospital with normal hemoglobin values went on to develop hospital-acquired anemia.[6] Of those admitted to the intensive care unit (ICU), 60% to 66% are anemic; by ICU day 8, 97% are anemic.[7] Surgical procedures, coagulation disorders, inflammation, renal failure, gastrointestinal bleeding, and phlebotomy are all causal factors in the development of iatrogenic anemia, as well as a variety of comorbid conditions (**Table 1**).

Box 1
Tenets of patient blood management

Rights to transfusion: right patient, right blood product, right indication, right time, right dose

Blood loss management

Identification and management of coagulopathies, including preventative assessments

Minimize iatrogenic blood loss

Blood-sparing modalities

Pharmaceuticals

Anemia management

Fluid therapy

Oxygen therapy

Box 2
Blood transfusion considerations and patient blood management care planning

- Timing of decision: emergent, urgent, or elective
- Informed patient ability for shared decision-making
- Are there alternative or adjuncts to transfusion therapy?
- Is there a disruption in oxygen delivery or oxygen carrying capacity? Most effective manner to correct
- Can there be a disruption in capillary bed functionality?
- Is anemia acute or chronic? Macrocirculation and microcirculation adaption
- Are there coexisting nutritional deficiencies?
- Acute blood loss, risk of rebleeding
- Hemodynamic stability
- Comorbidities
- Clotting factor deficiency, either genetic or acquired
- Ability to minimize or avoid risk
- Financial implications

Inflammatory states and hepcidin production are chief contributors in the development of anemia in chronic and critical illness, affecting RBC production in the following ways:

- Iron sequestration (inability to release and use iron)
- Blunted production of erythropoietin (EPO)
- Cytokine release resulting in reduced renal EPO production
- Macrophage activation of RBC destruction
- Diminished sensitivity of bone marrow receptors to EPO.

Table 1
Anemia in the critically ill

Type	Causes
Blood loss	Excessive phlebotomy Surgery Trauma Gastrointestinal bleeding
Coagulopathy	Thrombocytopenia Sepsis Hepatic disease or failure Splenomegaly Viral infection
Erythropoietin deficiencies	Anemia of chronic disease Inflammation Renal insufficiency or failure Endocrine disorders Infection
Nutritional deficiencies	Iron Folate Vitamin B 12
Hemolysis	Drug-induced toxins

EPO, a hormone produced in the adult kidney, is essential in the production of RBCs. Kidney dysfunction, a common complication seen in the ICU population, suppresses the release of EPO, resulting in reduced RBC production.[8] Hepcidin, a peptide produced in the liver, is the principal regulator of iron metabolism. Elevated hepcidin levels, triggered by inflammation, reduce iron absorption in the intestines, thus increasing further iron sequestration.

Requisite and frequent phlebotomy has a direct impact in iatrogenic anemia. The average patient hospitalized in an ICU will lose approximately 41 mL of blood per day through phlebotomy alone. Patients with high acuity can lose much higher volumes, often exceeding the body's ability to replace the lost RBCs.[9] Arterial blood gases account for as much as 40% of all ordered laboratory tests and are the most frequently ordered laboratory test in the ICU. Patients with in-dwelling arterial catheters are phlebotomized twice as often. Those with either arterial or central venous in-dwelling catheters can amass 3 times the amount of blood loss through phlebotomy as those without in-dwelling catheters.[10] Daily RBC production in a healthy adult is estimated to be 0.25 mL/kg, totaling approximately one-half liter per week. High volumes of blood loss through phlebotomy can often exceed the body's ability to maintain blood counts within normal range.[7]

Methods to reduce iatrogenic blood loss caused by phlebotomy include

- Lower volume laboratory tubes
- Refraining from ordering serial laboratory draws
- Assess need for routine laboratory tests on a daily basis
- Point-of-care blood analysis
- Adding on tests
- Reducing or eliminating blood waste when drawing from arterial catheter by using a closed blood sampling device
- Removal of indwelling catheters as soon as possible
- Monitoring pulse oximetry and capnography in lieu of arterial blood gas monitoring.

Approaches to reduce hemorrhagic blood loss include early detection of bleeding with the use of continuous hemoglobin monitoring, correction of body temperature and acidosis, and administration of select of pharmacologic agents.[11]

FLUID MANAGEMENT

Fluid management continues to be the most pervasive therapy given to hospitalized patients. Practices can vary by provider, hospital, and geographic location. It is important to recognize that blood products are not equal to intravenous (IV) fluids. Blood products should be considered as living tissue and given appropriate deliberation. Recent research suggests that fluid therapy is similar to the prescribing of medications and should have defined indications, as well as specified type, dose, rate, and duration.[12] The purpose of fluid therapy is to support cardiac output, tissue perfusion, and oxygen delivery.

Intravascular fluid is the delivery system of oxygen to vital tissue and organs, as well as the removal system of metabolic by-products. When this delivery system becomes disrupted by diminished blood volume, the heralded effects are decreased cardiac output, changes in microvasculature, and increases in blood viscosity. To counteract these effects, it is important to respond by treating according to the intended outcome. For example, if increasing cardiac output is the goal for hypovolemia, administering RBCs will not deliver. Adding cellular tissue will further increase blood viscosity and has been demonstrated to cause microvascular occlusion, further exacerbating oxygen delivery.[13] However, administering a balanced IV solution can fill the vascular space, decrease viscosity, and increase oxygen delivery.

Detrimental effects can occur from fluid therapy and these potential effects can determine which fluid is prescribed for a specific patient. There are 4 primary side effects to fluid therapy: hyperchloremic metabolic acidosis, hypocoagulopathy or hypercoagulopathy, impaired kidney function, and allergic reactions. Hyperchloremic metabolic acidosis results from an increase of chloride in plasma. It can be avoided by using IV fluids that do not have high chloride content, such as normal saline. IV fluids have the potential to dilute clotting factors. Crystalloid solutions can cause a mild hypercoagulopathy and albumin has been found to have an anticoagulation effect.[14]

There is no universal fluid that is applicable in all situations. When tissue perfusion is the goal, balanced crystalloid solutions are the best choice. To correct dehydration, the indicated solution is isotonic saline. In situations of significant blood loss, a noncalcium-containing balanced crystalloid can be used that will decrease the risk of hyperkalemia associated with administration of saline.[15]

PHARMACEUTICALS

Critically ill patients experience states of inflammation, immune system impairment, and nutritional deficiencies.[16] Nutritional and pharmaceutical support is used to provide essential nutrients and trace elements. Pharmaceuticals are available to stimulate the growth of blood cells, as well as to stop bleeding and manage coagulopathies (see later discussion). A study published in 2014 demonstrated that the degree of anemia at discharge can increase the risk for readmission.[17] Pharmaceutical treatments for anemia take time to work and do not provide rapid results. Therefore, these agents should be evaluated as preventative treatments, as well as for benefit beyond the intensive care setting. **Table 2** demonstrates the variety of agents available.

Iron deficiency and iron-restricted erythropoiesis is common in critical illness. The use of iron supplementation has been studied with varied findings of risk and benefits. A recent meta-analysis concluded that iron supplementation does not decrease RBC transfusions in intensive care patients; however, limitations included heterogeneity between comparison trials.[18] Notwithstanding this conclusion, there are equal studies and articles describing iron supplementation as a means to reduce transfusion requirements and manage anemia in critical care.[19,20] A previous meta-analysis found benefit in the use IV iron in reducing transfusion requirements and suggested wide application in acute care settings.[21] Just as confusing, is the literature regarding the propensity of IV iron to increase the risk of nosocomial infections. Consideration for the use of IV iron in the ICU setting include evaluation of pre-ICU risk factors or evidence of iron deficiency, current contraindications, and assessment of potential current and future benefits.

Vitamins and minerals essential for production of RBCs and the prevention of hemorrhage include B6, B12, vitamin C, vitamin E, and folic acid. Additional vitamin deficiencies can occur in certain patient populations, such as pregnant women, elderly, malnourished, and those with the medical conditions of renal failure and inflammatory bowel disease. Prevention is the best course of action in high prevalent groups.[22]

Cellular growth factors for RBCs have undergone study in the ICU environment primarily due to the finding that this patient population experiences blunted EPO response to anemia. There have been favorable conclusions in reduction of transfusion requirements; however, negative outcomes in terms of increased thrombotic

Table 2
Pharmaceutical alternatives

Agent	Indications	Dosage	References
IV iron (iron sucrose, ferric carboxymaltose, ferumoxytol)	Iron deficiency or depletion, impaired absorption, bleeding	Total combined dosing of 1000 mg to 1500 mg	Schrier et al,[39] 2016
Folic acid	Megaloblastic anemia, nutritional deficiency	Up to 1 mg/d Maintenance 0.4 mg	Drugs.com[40]
Vitamin B-12	Vitamin B12 deficiency, megaloblastic anemia	1 mg IM 3 times a week for 2 wk, then once every 3 mo	Romain et al,[41] 2016
Vitamin C	Low levels of vitamin C, increase demand, increase absorption of iron	100–1000 mg daily, depending on indication (oral)	National Institutes of Health[42] Mayo Clinic[44]
EPO	Stimulate RBC growth, chronic kidney disease, anemia of AIDS, anemia caused by chemotherapy	150–300 U/kg weekly or up to 3 times/wk	Drugs.com[45]
Granulocyte-colony stimulating factor (neupogen)	Stimulate granulocytes, risk of neutropenic fever of 20% or greater	5 μg/kg/d (filgrastim) 250 μg/m2 (sargramostim)	Larson et al,[43] 2016
Recombinant stem-cell factor (stemgen)	Shown to synergize with filgrastim to increase the number and mobilization of peripheral blood progenitor cells	20 μg/kg/d in conjunction with filgrastim	Medscape.com[46]
Vitamin K	Warfarin reversal	2.5–5 mg orally 10 mg IV infusion	Drugs.com[47]
Recombinant factor V11a	Massive transfusion associated with hypothermia, hyperfibrinolysis, dilutional coagulopathy, thrombocytopenia, and citrate excess with relative calcium deficiency Used to manage intractable nonsurgical bleeding that is unresponsive to routine hemostatic therapy	90 mg/kg every 2 h until hemostasis or treatment deemed inadequate Off-label use for patients without hemophilia	Shord & Lindley,[48] 2000
Recombinant factor IX	Surgical prophylaxis and severe bleeding prophylaxis in high-risk, patients Unable to accept primary transfusion components for religious reasons	Compute for desired effect	Shord & Lindley,[48] 2000

(continued on next page)

Table 2
(continued)

Agent	Indications	Dosage	References
Desmopressin (Ddavp)	Uremia, cirrhosis, prolonged cardiopulmonary bypass, antiplatelet drugs	4 μg/mL IV administered at 0.3 μg/kg	Drugs.com[49] Arthur,[50] 2013
E-aminocaproic acid (amicar)	Acute bleeding syndromes due to elevated fibrinolytic activity	16–20 mL (4–5 g)	Archived drug label, 2007[52]
Tranexamic acid (cyklokapron)	Cardiac surgery, GI bleeding, oral surgery, transurethral prostatectomy, liver transplant, multiple trauma, acute leukemia, postpartum hemorrhage	Varies by indication; IV and oral regimens	Shander & Seeber,[51] 2013
Conjugated estrogens	Abnormal uterine bleeding	25 mg IV, IM	Shander & Seeber,[51] 2013

Abbreviations: AIDS, acquired immune deficiency syndrome; GI, gastrointestinal; IM, intramuscular.
Data from Refs.[39–52]

events have also occurred. EPO is costly, carries a black box warning, has a delayed response, and depends on adequate iron availability, negating generalized use.[19,23] In 2012, a paper was published that evaluated available studies, including limitations and heterogeneity between studies, describing the lack of supporting data for use in critically ill patients.[24] The investigators suggested that the reduction in transfusion triggers have most likely nullified the primary endpoint of decreased transfusion requirements. The drug can be warranted in patients in whom blood transfusion is not an option or as continuation of therapy for chronic kidney disease. When using EPO it is important to ensure that the patient is not iron deficient and to monitor patient response through the assessment of reticulocyte counts.

HEMOSTATIC AGENTS

Coagulopathies in critically ill patients is common and often results from multiple factors. These include thrombocytopenia, disseminated intravascular coagulation, and prolonged clotting tests, as well as deficiencies and impairments of the clotting cascade.[25] A variety of hemostatic methods and agents are available to aid in the treatment of bleeding episodes and improving a patients' recovery or survival; however, management should be targeted toward the underlying condition. Health care providers may use platelets, plasma, or cryoprecipitate, either prophylactically or during acute bleeding episodes, without the benefit of high-quality studies supporting their use. Prophylactic use of plasma and platelets has not demonstrated patient benefit and can place patients a risk. Overuse of plasma can place patients at risk for mortality, infection, lung injury, and organ failure.[26,27]

There are laboratory tests and equipment to measure platelet function, clotting times, clot formation, and clot strength, each with its own limitations. These devices and equipment provide more definitive clinical data on which to base treatment decisions and have been shown to decrease the use of blood products. Point-of-care devices that can deliver results in less time paired with evidence-based algorithms have been demonstrated in multiple studies to reduce blood transfusions and decrease cost.[28]

In a health care landscape in which managing costs is at the forefront, many of these products have significant costs associated with them; therefore, it is important to weigh benefit, risks, and overall cost. Development of a program to serve as a clinical surveillance and management service has been shown to improve patient quality and lower costs associated with product usage. The concept is similar to what many hospitals have done with antimicrobial management initiatives. One hospital found that electronic restrictions did not achieve desirable outcomes in the diagnosing and use of these agents. Therefore, a team was assembled to aid in management of specific groups of patients using hemostatic agents: heparin-induced thrombocytopenia, hemophilia A or B, anticoagulation in patients on extracorporeal membrane oxygenation, and anticoagulation in patients with mechanical circulatory support. The results were impressive, including agent total dose reductions, decreased cost per patient day, and a total economic impact of 8 times the expense to run the program.[29]

MANUFACTURED BLOOD

The complexity of blood is reflected in the quest for blood substitutes and the manufacturing of products that can function to deliver oxygen. The concept has been derived to mitigate limitations and risks of human blood. Artificial blood would be disease free, have better oxygen transport capacity than banked blood, have a long shelf-life, eliminate cross-matching, excreted without damaging or taxing the kidneys, and would not induce untoward physiologic response.[30] Several decades of product development and research have yielded significant knowledge and progress toward the manufacturing of products. Product development and clinical trials have brought up safety concerns and issues with adverse events. Two groups of artificial oxygen carriers have emerged: (1) hemoglobin-based, either human or recombinant, and (2) perfluorocarbons, which are gases that develop during aluminum production. A third option has emerged in the engineering of RBCs via stem cell cultures.

A meta-analysis published in 2008 brought into question the safety of all hemoglobin-based oxygen carriers (HBOCs).[30] Evaluation of risk versus benefit of these products revolves around the question of their indication. Should they be considered as a replacement for allogeneic red cell transfusions or should they be used only when blood transfusion is not an option or is not available? Delineation of indication changes acceptable risk and tolerance of both serious and nonserious side effects. Van Hemeirijck and colleagues[31] (2014) conducted the only study comparing RBCs to HBOC-201 (OPK Biotech LLC, Cambridge, MA) with a primary endpoint of determining if the product could satisfy transfusion requirements without the need for allogeneic transfusions. Findings demonstrated that 43% of subjects treated with HBOC-201 avoided RBC transfusion without remarkable differences in mortality or serious adverse events when compared with a cohort with RBC transfusion. HBOC-201, or Hemopure, was approved for use in South Africa in 2001 but is restricted to investigational status in the United States by the Federal Drug Administration (FDA) primarily due to safety concerns. This product can be used for emergency or compassionate use only, which is based on individual request by a treating physician. A request can be made to the manufacturer and, if deemed appropriate, Biotech will notify the FDA for a single patient investigational new drug consent. A case study reported that more than 50 such approvals have been granted.[32]

A more recent product currently engaged in investigational trials is Sanguinate or pegylated bovine carboxyhemoglobin (PEG-HbCO; Prolong Pharmaceuticals, South Plainfield, NJ), which is attributed with delivering oxygen at the tissue or cellular level. This product has several phase II trials and has been designated as an orphan drug for sickle cell comorbidities. There is a phase I safety trial for patients with acute severe anemia in progress. In 2015, an abstract reported clinical improvement in a small cohort of 5 subjects receiving PEG-HbCO who could not receive transfusions either for religious beliefs or hemolytic reactions.[33] Findings from phase trials will determine future clinical applications.

Engineering red cells from stem cells has a role in worldwide health care, which is to meet needs of massive supply, rare blood groups, and the highest potential in the developing world. Progress has been made in how to culture red cells; however, challenges exist in the technical aspects and the ability to do so at a reasonable cost. Exciting possibilities exist for potential clinical applications of tissue-engineered RBCs. Two areas are drug discovery and drug delivery. Although considerable progress has been made, major challenges still need to be resolved. The future of this technology, as well as the other manufactured blood products, presents the possibility of future transformations in transfusion medicine.[34]

WHEN BLOOD IS NOT AN OPTION

In the event the patient refuses blood transfusion for personal or religious reasons, or has multiple antibodies (alloimmunization) limiting the availability of compatible blood products, interventions (**Table 3**) can be engaged to further minimize iatrogenic blood loss, stimulate red cell production, and prevent organ damage from critically low hemoglobin levels. Jehovah's Witnesses do not accept blood or the 4 primary components of blood (red cells, white cells, platelets, or plasma). Nor do they donate or store their own blood. The belief is derived from biblical interpretation that forbids the consumption of blood. However, some will accept fractions of blood as a personal choice. Blood fractions are derivatives extracted from the 4 primary blood components. Fractions obtained from hemoglobin (human or animal) have benefited patients who experience massive hemorrhage or acute anemia. Plasma fractions include proteins, clotting factors, and antibodies (albumin, gamma globulins). The avoidance of blood products by this group has led to advancements in the evidence surrounding the efficacy and effectiveness of conservative transfusion therapies and practice.[35,36]

Jehovah's Witnesses and others who refuse blood transfusion desire to receive care in a health care environment that is respectful of their beliefs. Such patients want to be assured that the health care team will use all available means for treatment without the

Table 3 Strategies to minimize blood loss	
General Strategies	**Therapeutic Principles**
Create a detailed and individualized clinical management plan to minimize blood loss and treat anemia	Proactive approaches to anticipate, prepare, and manage uncontrolled blood loss
Use a multidisciplinary team approach to clinical care	Preoperative workup
Early recognition of blood loss or physiologic deterioration	Management strategies to optimize patients preoperatively
Promptly act to maintain hemostasis in the actively bleeding patient by using testing that provides rapid results and minimizes delays	Restrict phlebotomy
Be prepared to modify routine practice	Meticulous surgical hemostasis Optimize oxygen delivery Minimize oxygen consumption

use of blood. Communication is extremely important in these situations. Measures should be taken to ensure that communication is free from coercion from the health care team. It is recommended that a communication approach is established between the health care team and the patient or family:

- Identify member or members of the health care team that will be responsible for communication
- Identify patient surrogate if the patient is unable
- Establish communication boundaries.

There is a legal and moral requirement to provide the opportunity to change decision regarding blood products. It should be stressed that when discussing blood transfusion care should be taken so the discussion is not perceived as coercion. Dialogue should occur daily during periods of critical illness or when changes in status occur, with an emphasis that treatments are being implemented and what can be done within the parameters of treatment acceptable to the patient.[37]

Preventative measures should be used when risk of severe anemia is present. When critical anemia occurs, having a protocol available will provide guidance and a framework for patient management. Criteria for protocol execution should be massive blood loss and/or hemoglobin levels below 5 gm/dL. It is also important to create a knowledgeable team during critical anemia by consulting a hospital blood management team (if available), hematology, or Jehovah's Witness hospital liaison committee member or minister.

Repeated exposure by frequent blood transfusion and pregnancy can be associated with increased rates of alloimmunization. Described as an immune response caused by incompatibility between donor and recipient antigens, it is most often seen in individuals with disorders requiring chronic transfusion (sickle cell disease, thalassemia) and women who are pregnant. Alloimmunity can result in dire consequences for the fetus (death) or the inability to locate compatible blood. If transfusion of the alloimmunized patient is anticipated, the hospital blood bank should be notified as soon as possible to allow time to locate compatible blood. For rare blood, a local, regional, and sometimes national search for compatible blood should be initiated. Interventions listed in **Table 4** may also be used as a bridge to transfusion until compatible blood is located.[38]

Whether blood is not an option due to religious or personal reasons, or due to limited or unavailability of compatible blood, interventions to manage critical anemia or active bleeding are vital. It is crucial to support the cardiovascular system, maximize oxygenation, reduce oxygen consumption, reduce or eliminate further blood loss, and stimulate RBC production (**Table 5**).

Table 4
Jehovah's Witness position on blood and blood fractions

Jehovah's Witnesses' Basic Position on Blood				
Not acceptable (whole blood)	Red cells	White cells	Plasma	Platelets
Personal decision	Red cell fractions • Hemoglobin-based blood substitutes	White cell fractions • Interferons • Interleukin	Plasma fractions • Albumin • Globulins • Clotting factors • Cryoprecipitate	Platelet fractions • Wound healing factor

Table 5 Critical anemia	
Active Bleeding	**Critical Anemia Hgb <5 gm/dL**
Cautious fluid resuscitation	IV iron
Emergent surgical interventions	• Administer daily in divided doses up to 1 gm then
Cryoprecipitate	re-evaluate
Vitamin K	Procrit (preferred due to response onset, contains
Factor concentrates	albumin)
IV iron	• 40,000 units SQ every other day for 1 wk OR
Procrit 40,000 units SQ	• 20,000 units SQ daily for 3 d (recommended for
Prothrombin concentrates	nonbleeding)
Intraoperative measures	• May be given intravenously if necessary (SQ is
• Hemostatic agents	preferred route of administration)
• Cell salvage	Darbepoetin
• Normovolemic hemodilution	• 200 μg SQ once/wk OR
	• 100 μg SQ once/wk (recommend for nonbleeding)
	Monitor reticulocyte count to assess bone marrow
	response
	Darbepoetin does not use albumin as a carrier
	molecule
	Vitamin C 500 mg IV
	Vitamin B12 1000 μg IM or IV
	Folate 1 mg IV
	Pediatric blood tubes
	Point-of-care testing
	No routine blood draws
	Only essential laboratory work
	Noninvasive hemoglobin monitoring
	Minimize dressing changes to reduce blood loss
	Measures to reduce oxygen demand
	• Sedation
	• Mechanical ventilation
	• Neuromuscular blockade
	Maximize oxygen delivery
	• Supplemental O2
	• Hyperbaric therapy

Abbreviations: Hgb, hemoglobin; O2, oxygen; SQ, subcutaneous.

SUMMARY

Alternatives and adjuncts to blood transfusions are widely accessible and should be tailored to the specific needs of individual patients. Restrictive transfusion practices have been shown to be effective. Universally, critically ill patients should be transfused under current guidelines with simple blood management modalities, such as anemia tolerance, reduction in the amount of blood drawn for blood gases and laboratory testing, and fluid therapy. Additional considerations for blood products are attention to dosing, prescribing 1 unit of RBCs, and re-evaluating for the need of additional units. Hemostatic agents and pharmaceuticals may be of benefit; however, evidence and cost should be considered. When blood is not an option, preventative anemia treatment should begin early with the availability of critical anemia protocols. The overall conclusion is that there continues to be gaps in knowledge in the use of transfusion alternatives. Therefore, individual patient-specific treatment plans should be the desired goal.

REFERENCES

1. Cannon-Diebl MR. Transfusion in the critically ill: does it affect outcome? Crit Care Nurs Q 2010;35(4):324–38.
2. Shander A, Fink A, Javidroozi M, et al, International Consensus Conference on Transfusion Outcomes Group. Appropriateness of allogeneic red blood cell transfusion: the international consensus conference on transfusion outcomes. Transfus Med Rev 2011;25(3):232–46.e53.
3. AABB, American Red Cross, America's Blood Centers, and Armed Services Blood Program. Circular of information for the use of human blood and blood components. 2016. Available at: https://www.aabb.org/tm/coi/Documents/coi1113.pdf. Accessed September 20, 2016.
4. Callum L, Waters JH, Shaz BH, et al. The AABB recommendations for the Choosing Wisely campaign of the American Board of Internal Medicine. Transfusion 2014;54:2344–52.
5. Isbister JP. The three-pillar matrix of patient blood management: an overview. Best Pract Res Clin Anesthesiol 2013;27:69–84.
6. Koch C, Li L, Sun Z, et al. Hospital-acquired anemia: prevalence, outcomes, and healthcare implications. J Hosp Med 2015;8(9):506–12.
7. McEvoy M, Shander A. Anemia, bleeding, and blood transfusion in the intensive care unit: causes, risks, costs and new strategies. Am J Crit Care 2013;22(6):eS1–14.
8. Patel N, Collino M, Yaqoob M, et al. Erythropoietin in the intensive care unit: beyond treatment of anemia. Ann Intensive Care 2011;1:40.
9. Vincent J, Baron J, Reinhart K, et al. Anemia and blood transfusion in critically ill patients. JAMA 2002;288(12):1499–507.
10. Fowler R, Berenson M. Blood conversation in the intensive care unit. Crit Care Med 2003;31(12 Suppl):S715–20.
11. Patterson T, Stein M. Hemorrhage and coagulopathy in the critically ill. Emerg Med Clin North Am 2005;32(4):797–810. Available at: https://www.clinicalkey.com/#!/content/playContent/1-s2.0-S0733862714000601?returnurl=http:%2F%2Flinkinghub.elsevier.com%2Fretrieve%2Fpii%2FS0733862714000601%3Fshowall%3Dtrue&referrer. Accessed October 11, 2016.
12. Moritz M, Ayus JC. Maintenance intravenous fluids in acutely ill patients. N Engl J Med 2015;373:1350–60.
13. Orlov D, Karkouti K. The pathophysiology and consequences of red blood cell storage. Anesthesia 2015;70:29–37.
14. Seeber P, Shander A. Fluid therapy. In: Murphy MF, Roberts DJ, Yazer MH, editors. Basics of blood management. 2nd edition. West Sussex (United Kingdom): Wiley-Blackwell; 2013. p. 67–78.
15. Raghunathan K, Nailer P, Konoske R. What is the ideal crystalloid? Curr Opin Crit Care 2015;21:309–14.
16. Rech M, To L, Tovbin A, et al. Heavy metal in the intensive care unit: a review of current literature on trace element supplementation in critically ill patients. Nutr Clin Pract 2013;29:78–89.
17. Koch CG, Li L, Sun Z, et al. Magnitude of anemia at discharge increased 30-day hospital readmissions. J Patient Saf 2014 [Epub ahead of print]. Available at: journalofpatientsafety.com.
18. Shah A, Roy NB, McKechnie S, et al. Iron supplementation to treat anaemia in adult critical care patients: a systematic review and meta-analysis. Crit Care 2016;20:306.

19. Hayden JH, Albert TJ, Watkins TR, et al. Anemia in critical illness: insights into etiology, consequences, and management. Am J Respir Crit Care Med 2012;185: 1049–57.

20. Goddard AF, James MW, McIntyre AS, et al. Guidelines for the management of iron deficiency anaemia. Gut 2011;60:1309–16.

21. Litton E, Ziao J, Ho KM. Safety and efficacy of intravenous iron therapy in reducing requirement of allogeneic blood transfusion: systematic review and meta-analysis of randomized clinical trials. BMJ 2013;347:f4822.

22. Seeber P, Shander A. Anemia therapy II: hematinic. In: Basics of blood management. 2nd edition. West Sussex (United Kingdom): Wiley-Blackwell; 2013. p. 36–48.

23. Shermock KM, Rice TL. Erythropoietic agents for anemia of critical illness. Am J Health Syst Pharm 2008;15:540–6.

24. Piagnerelli M, Vincent JL. The use of erythropoiesis-stimulating agents in the intensive care unit. Crit Care Clin 2012;28:345–62.

25. Levi M, Opal SM. Coagulation abnormalities in critically ill patients. Crit Care 2006;10(4):222.

26. Mahambry T, Pendry K, Nee A, et al. Critical care in emergency department: massive haemorrhage in trauma. Emerg Med J 2013;30:9–14.

27. Spahn DR, Rossaint R. Coagulopathy and blood component transfusion in trauma. Br J Anesth 2005;95:130–9.

28. Theusinger OM, Stein P, Levy JH. Point of care and factor concentrate-based coagulation algorithms. Transfus Med Hemother 2015;42:115–21.

29. Reardon DP, Atay JK, Ashley SW, et al. Implementation of a hemostatic and antithrombotic stewardship program. J Thromb Thrombolysis 2015;40:379–82.

30. Bartlett R. Oxygen therapeutics: the quest for artificial blood. In: Jabbour N, editor. Transfusion free medicine and surgery. Malden (MA): Blackwell Publishing; 2005. p. XX.

31. Van Hemeirijck J, Levien LJ, Veeckman L, et al. A safety and efficacy evaluation of hemoglobin-based oxygen carrier HBOC-201 in a randomized, multicenter red blood cell controlled trial in noncardiac surgery patients. Anesth Analg 2014; 119(4):766–76.

32. Jordan SD, Alexander E. Bovine hemoglobin: a nontraditional approach to the management of acute anemia in a Jehovah's Witness patient with autoimmune hemolytic anemia. J Pharm Pract 2012;26(3):257–60.

33. Parmar DV, Misra HK, Berryman JB, et al. Potential use of PEG-HbCO in severe anemia. Abstract at 2015 ASCO Annual Meeting. J Clin Oncol 2015;33(Suppl) [abstract: e18086]. Available at: http://www.prolongpharma.com/asco-2015-publishes-prolong-pharmaceuticals-llcs-e-abstract-of-the-potential-use-of-peg-hbco-in-severe-anemia-in-5-eind-patients/. Accessed September 29, 2016.

34. Van Heen T, Hunt JA. Tissue engineering red blood cells: a therapeutic. J Tissue Eng Regen Med 2015;9:760–70.

35. Weiss G, Goodnough L. Anemia of chronic disease. N Engl J Med 2005;352(10): 11–23. Available at: http://www.med.unc.edu/medclerk/medselect/files/anemia2. pdf. Accessed October 10, 2016.

36. Watchtower ONLINE LIBRARY. Keep yourselves in God's love. Blood fractions and surgical procedures. Appendix. 2016;215–216. Available at: http://wol.jw. org/en/wol/d/r1/lp-e/1102008086. Accessed October 18, 2016.

37. West J. Ethical issues in the care of Jehovah's Witnesses. Curr Opin Anesthesiol 2014;27(2):170–6.

38. Nance S. Management of alloimmunized patients. International Society of Blood Transfusion. ISBT Sci Ser 2010;5:274–8. Available at: http://onlinelibrary.wiley.com/doi/10.1111/j.1751-2824.2010.01381.x/epdf. Accessed October 18, 2016.

39. Schrier SL, Auerbach M, Mentzer WC, et al. Treatment of iron deficiency anemia in adults. 2016. Available at: https://www.uptodate.com/contents/treatment-of-iron-deficiency-anemia-in-adults. Accessed October 18, 2016.

40. Drugs.com. Folic acid. Available at: https://www.drugs.com/pro/folic-acid.html. Accessed October 18, 2016.

41. Romain M, Sviri S, Linton DM, et al. The role of vitamin B12 in the critically ill: a review. Anesthes Intensive Care 2016;44:447–52.

42. National Institutes of Health. Vitamin C: fact sheet for health professionals. 2016. Available at: https://ods.od.nih.gov/factsheets/VitaminC-HealthProfessional/. Accessed October 18, 2016.

43. Larson RA, Drews RE, Savarese DM. Use of granulocyte colony stimulating factors in adults patients with chemotherapy-induced neutropenia and conditions other than acute leukemia, myelodysplastic syndrome, and hematopoietic cell transplantation. Available at: https://www.uptodate.com/contents/use-of-granulocyte-colony-stimulating-factors-in-adult-patients-with-chemotherapy-induced-neutropenia-and-conditions-other-than-acute-leukemia-myelodysplastic-syndrome-and-hematopoietic-cell-transplantation#H523774247. Accessed October 18, 2016.

44. Mayo Clinic. Vitamin C (ascorbic acid). Available at: http://www.mayoclinic.org/drugs-supplements/vitamin-c/dosing/hrb-20060322. Accessed October 18, 2016.

45. Drugs.com. Erythropoietin. Available at: https://www.drugs.com/search.php?searchterm=erythropoietin&a=1. Accessed October 18, 2016.

46. Medscape.com. Stemgen. Available at: http://reference.medscape.come/drug/stemgen-ancestim-342267. Accessed October 19, 2016.

47. Drugs.com. Vitamin K. Available at: https://www.drugs.com/search.php?searchterm=Vitamin+C. Accessed October 28, 2016.

48. Shord S, Lindley CM. Coagulation products and their uses. Am J Health Syst Pharm 2000;57(15):1403–17.

49. Drugs.com. Desmopressin. Available at: https://www.drugs.com/monograph/factor-ix-recombinant.html 10/19/2016. Accessed October 19, 2016.

50. Arthur M. Bloodless medicine: available alternative to transfusions in cardiac surgery. 2013. Available at: http://www.augusta.edu/mcg/anes/clinical-specialities/documents/arthur_bloodless-medicine0213.pdf. Accessed October 19, 2016.

51. Seeber P, Shander A. Basics of blood management. 2nd edition. West Sussex (United Kingdom): Wiley-Blackwell; 2013. p. 82–8.

52. Archived drug label. Aminocaproic acid. Available at: https://dailymed.nim.nih.gov/dailymed/archieves/fdadruginfol.cfm?archieveid=5242. Accessed October 19, 2016.

The Risks Associated with Red Blood Cell Transfusion

Implications for Critical Care Practice

Douglas H. Sutton, EdD, MSN, MPA, APRN, NP-C[a],*,
Deborah A. Raines, PhD, EDS, RN, ANEF[b]

KEYWORDS

- Blood transfusion • Complications of transfusions
- Critical care blood replacement intervention

KEY POINTS

- Blood replacement is a common intervention in critical care settings.
- Blood replacement is not without risk and may increase morbidity and mortality in critically ill patients.
- Symptomatic replacement may warrant further consideration, versus relying solely on physiologic data.
- Blood replacement may have greater risk than benefit in certain clinical conditions and in different age groups.

INTRODUCTION

Anemia is among most common abnormal laboratory finding in the population of critically ill patients. Approximately 95% of patients in the intensive care unit (ICU) for 3 days or more are anemic, and approximately 50% of these patients receive an average of 5 units of packed red blood cells (PRBCs) while in the ICU.[1,2] Many of these transfusions are given to treat a low hemoglobin, not active bleeding. In the past, anemia was thought to lead to increased morbidity and mortality in the critically ill patient and transfusion with PRBCs was often implemented to maintain a preillness blood value to prevent morbidity and mortality. However, whether the increased morbidity and mortality seen in the ICU population is related to the anemic state or more severe disease process is not clearly explicated.[3] Traditionally, the goal of administering PRBCs to the critically ill patient was to increase hemoglobin levels, to improve the blood's oxygen carrying

The authors have nothing to disclose.
[a] College of Health and Human Services, Northern Arizona University, 2065 West Dolores Lane, Flagstaff, AZ 86005, USA; [b] School of Nursing, University at Buffalo, 3435 Main Street, Buffalo, NY 14214-3079, USA
* Corresponding author.
E-mail address: douglas.sutton@nau.edu

capacity, and to oxygenate hypoxic tissue. However, an emerging body of evidence is demonstrating that this clinical benefit is often not achieved.

In patients with active bleeding or hemorrhage, PRBC transfusion can be a life-saving intervention. With acute blood loss, transfusion of PRBCs can increase arterial oxygen content and cardiac output. However, understanding the mechanism of anemia in the critically ill population, in the absence of active blood loss, is more complex and multifactorial. These factors include multiple phlebotomies, nutritional deficiencies and decreased erythropoietin production. Critical illness alone mediates a decrease in red blood cell (RBC) mass, leading to anemia. This effect is mediated by a variety of inflammatory cytokines such as interleukin-1 and tumor necrosis factor-alpha, which inhibit erythropoietin production and lower the rate of RBC production. As a result of lowered rate of production and increased iatrogenic loss through frequent phlebotomy, hemoglobin levels decrease.[2] Some decrease in hematocrit may be beneficial in the critically ill patient because the decrease in viscosity may increase oxygen availability to the cell by improving the flow of blood in the microcirculation. Consequently, the transfusion of PRBCs to increase the hemoglobin concentration, which increases the oxygen-carrying capacity of the blood could very well be offset by a decrease in cardiac output because of the increase in blood viscosity associated with a decreased sympathetic response. Thus, blood transfusion in the critically ill population, in the absence of active bleeding, may increase morbidity and mortality among critically ill patients. This systematic review is designed to answer the question, in the critically ill patient who is not actively bleeding, is the transfusion of a single unit of PRBCs helpful or harmful?

METHOD
Study Design

The need for scientific evidence to determine best practices is essential to safe, quality patient care. This systematic review followed the methodological standards recommended by the Preferred Reporting Items for Systematic Reviews and Meta-Analysis (PRISMA) Statement.[4] The purpose was to identify, evaluate, and synthesize empirical evidence to answer the question, "In the critically ill patient who is not actively bleeding, is the transfusion of a single unit of PRBC helpful or harmful?" A systematic review presents a synthesis of the evidence from which conclusions can be drawn to make informed decisions about best practices in the patient care setting.[5]

Search Criteria

A search was conducted to identify empiric evidence related to the benefit or harm of transfusion of PRBCs in the critically ill population, in the absence of active bleeding. An electronic search followed by a manual search and screen was conducted. The electronic databases used for this review included PubMed, CINHAL, Cochrane, MedLine, Scopus, BMJ Clinical Evidence, and Web of Science. The search strategy was constrained to empirical studies on critically ill patients of any age in hospital settings and receiving at least a single PRBC transfusion. Studies published between 2008 and 2016 were included. The review did not exclude studies based on language. A manual search of the reference lists of the published articles was conducted to identify additional eligible studies for review. Manual screening of published articles was conducted to verify the empiric evidence was clinically appropriate and specific to the critically ill population.

Search terms included the keywords blood, blood products, adverse blood transfusion reactions, risk factors and blood transfusion, side effects of blood products, and blood transfusions and critical OR emergency care. To get relevant articles, the

Boolean operators "AND" and "OR" were also used. Thus, the search term involved blood products transfusion "AND" critical care practice, side effects of blood products "AND" critical care practice "OR" blood transfusions reactions in critically ill patients. A total of 372 studies were retrieved.

Study Selection

Copies of the titles and abstracts, when available, of the identified studies (N = 372), were obtained. The screening process eliminated duplicate articles (N = 6) and articles with irrelevant outcomes (N = 353). Criteria for irrelevant outcomes included transfusion in a situation with active bleeding, noncritically ill population, or use of volume replacement other than blood product transfusion. Thirteen studies remained. Full-text copies of these studies were obtained for further review. One article (N = 1) was excluded because the outcome was not considered eligible for inclusion, 2 articles (N = 2) were found to be duplicated. The remaining 10 studies were selected for inclusion in this review. The PRISMA flowchart illustrating the selection process is shown in **Fig. 1**.

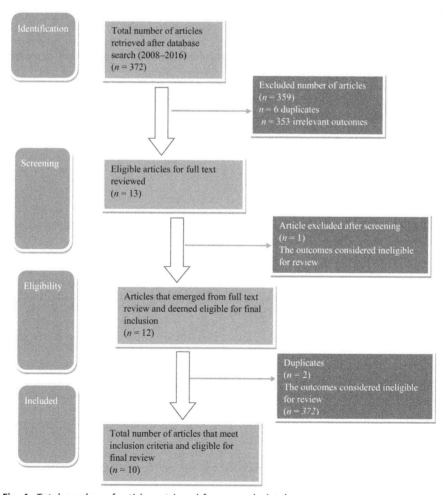

Fig. 1. Total number of articles retrieved from search databases.

Data extraction and assessment of risk of bias
Data were mined from all the included studies. The study characteristics extracted included design, setting (ie, clinical setting and country), sample size, and variable and key findings. The literature matrix is shown in **Table 1**.

To assess the risk of bias, the Cochrane Risk of Bias Tool was used because it provided the domains of random sequence generation. The components of the risk of bias were rated as "yes," "probably yes" (to show a low risk of bias), "probably no," and "no" show a higher risk of bias. If the responses are "no," or "probably no" for the random sequence generation, this was considered a higher risk of bias.[5]

Presentation of Eligible Articles

The articles that were eligible included randomized controlled trials (RCTs), a retrospective cohort study, and a prospective observational study. These studies involved subjects receiving a single unit of blood or PRBCs The RCTs were performed among subjects who received at least a single unit of blood or PRBCs. Other studies only mentioned that the subjects were given a single unit blood transfusion in the ICU. Subjects were randomly selected and assigned to the liberal practice of blood transfusion. The outcome measures included mortality and morbidity regarding acute respiratory distress syndrome, acute renal injury, and cardiogenic shock. The clinical settings included preoperative and postoperative critical care settings. There were no restrictions and participants of all age groups were included. The subjects were recruited from health care settings with a focus on those admitted to the critical care unit. Follow-up of the admitted subjects was done from the time of their admission to the ICU until discharge from the hospital. All the studies were carried out to evaluate the risk and implications of receiving at least a single unit blood transfusion in intensive or critical care practice. The eligible articles were compared based on their research findings as presented in **Table 1**, which summarizes the characteristics of eligible articles included in the review.

QUALITATIVE ANALYSIS

After analyzing the various heterogeneous study designs included in this systematic review, it becomes apparent that there are few RCTs that have investigated the risks associated with a critically ill patient receiving a single unit PRBC transfusion. It is widely reported that well designed and executed RCTs provide the most reliable evidence for inclusion in systematic reviews. Therefore, the data available did not allow the authors the ability to use formal statistical analysis to conduct a meta-analysis. Instead, each study was evaluated concerning the strength and generalizability based on the context of the study.

RESULTS

Ten studies met the selection criteria. The studies examined the effects of transfusing a single unit of PRBCs in the critically ill subject. Most of the study designs included in this systematic review of the literature were either retrospective or prospective, and only 1 was a randomized controlled study. A common finding among all studies was that transfusion of a single unit of PRBCs in the critically ill subject increases risk and may lead to increased morbidity and mortality. The table lists the studies and their key findings.

The studies relied on biophysical data to ascertain risk associated with PRBC transfusion. Firm conclusions are limited due to either study design. However, sample size for all included studies was adequate for the statistical methodology used to analyze results. Based on these findings, it seems that all included studies identified some risk associated with the transfusion of a single unit of PRBCs in the critically ill patient. Following careful analysis of the subject outcomes from each of the included studies, the following 4 primary clinical findings categories were formulated:

1. No increased risk in single versus double transfused PRBCs
2. Risk increases as the number of transfused PRBCs increases
3. Immune changes due to transfusion of PRBCs
4. Patient survival following a transfusion of PRBCs.

Berger and colleagues,[6] reported that overall survival of critically ill chemotherapy or stem cell transplant survivors experienced a similar survival rate in single-unit versus double-unit PRBC transfusion. Hajjar and colleagues[7] reported that subjects who undergo cardiac surgery, and who have a restrictive protocol versus a liberal protocol for administering PRBC transfusion, experience the same 30-day all-cause mortality rate. Szpila and colleagues[8] reported that in the surgical intensive care setting a restrictive transfusion protocol did not result in a change in morbidity or mortality for this subject population. Finally, Toy and colleagues[9] reported that transfusion was not found to be a significant risk for transfusion-related acute lung injury. Each of these studies, although all conducted on critically ill subjects with various diagnoses, revealed that there were no statistically significant differences in reported complications or changes in morbidity and mortality.

Dos Santos and colleagues[10] reported that, in subjects who undergo a coronary artery bypass graft (CABG) procedure, there is a dose-dependent relationship between the number of transfused PRBCs and mortality risk. Rubinstein and colleagues[11] evaluated data on 12,971 subjects who had undergone a carotid endarterectomy (CEA) procedure and discovered that subjects who received even 1 unit of transfused PRBCs have a 5-fold increase in stroke risk secondary to an inflammatory and hypercoagulable reaction. Whitlock and Auerbach,[12] in their retrospective study of 1,583,819 records of patients who had not undergone cardiac, intracranial, or vascular procedures, found that these critically ill patients were still at increased risk of experiencing an ischemic stroke or myocardial infarction. Each of these studies identified instances of increased risk associated with receiving transfused PRBCs.

Four of the included studies identified at least some alteration in the physiologic immune response in relation to receiving a transfusion of PRBCs. Christou and colleagues[13] reported that transfusion of PRBCs enhances the formation of allergenic RBCs, which heightens the risk of the subject experiencing immunologic incompatibility with subsequent transfusions. Kumar and colleagues[14] reported that 225 acute reactions occurred in 21,971 transfusions. Of these, febrile nonhemolytic transfusion reactions accounted for 60.4%, allergic reactions 31.2%, hemolytic reactions 0.4%, and nonspecific reactions 8%. The investigators highlight the need for clinicians to be better aware of transfusion reactions because these may be underreported in critically ill clients due to confounding physiologic alterations related to the primary admission diagnosis. Rubinstein and colleagues[11] reported that, in subjects who had undergone a CEA surgical procedure, and who receive an erythrocyte transfusion, the immune system initiates an inflammatory response, which results in a state of hypercoagulability, which increases the risk of stroke. Zalpuri and colleagues[15] report similar findings to other studies in which they conclude that transfusion of a single unit of PRBCs suppresses the immune system and that the physiologic insult triggers an immune response similar to what Rubinstein and colleagues[11] reported in their conclusions.

Table 1
Characteristics of included trials on the risk of a single-unit blood transfusion and the implications in critical care practice

Source	Design	Setting	Sample	Variable	Findings
Berger et al,[6] 2012	Retrospective cohort	ICU Switzerland	139 subjects receiving intensive chemotherapy or stem cell transplantation	PRBC transfusion	A single-unit blood transfusion led to a 25% reduction of RBC usage per treatment cycle with chemotherapy but was not associated with higher outpatient transfusion frequency There was no evidence of more severe bleeding or more platelet transfusions in single vs double unit transfusions Overall survival between single-unit and double-unit transfusions were similar in both cohorts
Christou et al,[13] 2013	Prospective Descriptive	ICU Canada	17 subjects	PRBC transfusion	No significant difference was found in the number of vascular progenitor cells between transfused and nontransfused subjects Transfusion enhances the formation of allergenic RBCs, which contributes to immunologic incompatibility
Dos Santos et al,[10] 2013	Retrospective comparative	ICU Brazil	3010 subjects undergoing CABG	PRBC transfusion	There is a dose-dependent relationship between the number of PBRCs transfused and mortality risk in subjects who have undergone CABG
Hajjar et al,[7] 2010	Prospective RCT	ICU Brazil	512 subjects Scheduled for cardiac surgery	PRBC transfusion protocol: liberal vs restrictive	In subjects undergoing cardiac surgery, there was no difference in the rate of 30-d all-cause mortality and severe mortality based on the assigned protocol for administering a PRBC transfusion
Kumar et al,[14] 2014	Retrospective Descriptive	Critical care units India	21,971 blood components were administered in ICU	Acute transfusion reactions	225 acute transfusion reactions (ATRs) were reported The frequency of ATR occurrence was: febrile nonhemolytic transfusion reactions (FNHTR) 136 (60.4%), allergic reactions 70 (31.2%), hemolytic reactions 1 (0.4%), and nonspecific reactions 18 (8%) Consideration of the deleterious effects of blood products can decrease transfusion-related morbidity and mortality in the critically ill population

Study	Study Design	Setting / Location	Subjects	Intervention	Findings
Rubinstein et al,[11] 2013	Prospective cohort	ICU United States	12,786 subjects with carotid endarterectomy (CEA)	1–2 unit PRBC transfusion	Transfusion of 1 unit of PBRCs resulted in a 5-fold increase in stroke risk due to inflammatory and hypercoagulable reactions provoked by erythrocyte transfusion
Szpila et al,[8] 2015	Retrospective historical case-control	Surgical ICU subjects United States	829 subjects	PRBC and fresh frozen plasma transfusion protocol	A restrictive transfusion protocol in critically ill surgical subjects did not increase morbidity or mortality
Toy et al,[9] 2015	Prospective case control	ICU United States	308 subjects	PRBC transfusion	Transfusion was not found to be a significant risk factor for transfusion-related acute lung injury but, instead, the primary cause was associated with the recipients' acute respiratory distress syndrome risk factors and onset of new lung injury
Whitlock et al,[12] 2015	Retrospective cohort	346 hospital operating rooms United States	1,583,819 adults who underwent noncardiac, nonintracranial, nonvascular surgery	PRBC transfusion	A preoperative blood transfusion of 1 unit of PRBCs was associated with increased odds of ischemic stroke and myocardial infarction
Zalpuri et al,[15] 2014	Cohort	ICU Netherlands	5746 subjects	PRBC transfusion	Transfusion of a single unit of RBCs suppresses the immune system and can be a trigger in the development of an immune response Traumatic injury Transfusions can lead to microchimerism and lead to immunosuppression, predisposing the subject to a diminished alloantigenic response

Data from Refs.[6–15]

The final category of findings relates to survival outcomes in critically ill patients who have undergone a transfusion of PRBCs. Berger and colleagues[6] reported that subjects receiving intensive chemotherapy or who have undergone a stem cell transplant had overall survival rates similar regardless of whether they received single-unit versus double-unit transfusions of PRBCs. Christou and colleagues[13] reported that transfusion enhances the formation of allergenic RBCs, which contributes to subsequent immunologic incompatibility. As a result, depending on the physiologic response, patients may experience adverse outcomes related to future transfusions of PRBCs. Kumar and colleagues[14] recommend increased awareness and recognition of acute transfusion reactions (ATR) as a way to decrease mortality and morbidity in the critically ill patient.

Findings from these studies highlight the need for a judicious protocol related to transfusion of PRBCs. Also, consistent with these findings, is the conclusion that transfusion of erythrocytes comes with inherent risk. The body recognizes the foreign antigens and triggers an immune response and, depending on the baseline hemodynamic status of the critically ill patient, outcomes may be negatively affected related to actual morbidity and mortality. Finally, in certain populations of critically ill patients, the use of transfused PRBCs may be severely restricted. Patients who have undergone CABG or CEA are at especially high risk following transfusion of PRBCs.

Exposure to a single unit of transfused allogeneic PRBCs may lead to alloimmunization. It also may result in prolonged patient stays in ICUs, increased risk for the development of infections, and systemic inflammatory response syndrome.[15] In a study conducted in Ottawa, Canada, in subjects being cared for in the intensive care setting, those who received a transfusion with blood products such as RBCs, platelets, or plasma were more likely to require prolonged hospital length-of-stay and have a higher mortality rate than those who did not require a transfusion.[16]

DISCUSSION

The primary purpose of conducting a systematic review approach is to ensure that the best available knowledge on the topic was synthesized. The validation taken in each step while determining the eligible articles decreases the risk of bias as well as extraction errors during the review. The eligible studies provided convincing results on the risks associated with receiving a single transfusion of PRBCs in the critical care unit. Significant findings were obtained from the eligible results and it is evident that PRBC transfusion is an intervention that is not without inherent risk in the critically ill patient. The studies included were methodologically sound and the results consistently demonstrated a relationship between receiving a single transfusion of PRBCs and increased risk, primarily in the form of an immunologic change that occurs because of a foreign antigen response, resulting in increased mortality and morbidity for the critically ill patient. Higher mortality rates are also associated with patients with certain surgical diagnoses, such as CABG and CEA. One study found that there was a need for clinicians caring for critically ill patients to receive transfusion therapy to be better aware of ATRs that may be masked by the hemodynamic changes of the admitting diagnosis or surgical procedure. The investigators reported that, as a result of the subjects' severity of illness, ATRs are underreported in this population. The findings from each of the studies included demonstrate that there are significant risks when receiving RBC transfusion therapy.

The content and quality of the selected studies served as the foundation of presenting known risks associated with transfusion of PRBCs in the critically ill patient for this systematic review of the literature. Findings reveal that there is further need for more robust research related to blood transfusion as an intervention because it poses a significant risk for some patients as revealed in these systematic review conclusions. Study designs varied among the selected articles, with only 1 true RCT included that was based on the question, developed for this review of the literature. Although the selected studies were found to be comprehensive in design, only a single study met the scientific rigor of the RCT. Considering that transfusion of PRBCs is not a new intervention, this finding was unexpected. For the reader of this systematic review, this may lead to some skepticism regarding the reported outcomes. It would, therefore, be expected that the actual therapeutic benefit and risk associated with RBC transfusion therapy is yet not well understood.

The results of the studies included in this systematic review provide the current published evidence concerning potential clinical outcomes and complications associated with a single transfusion of PRBCs. The studies investigated the effects of RBC transfusion as an intervention for patients in the critical care setting and multiple studies reported the increased risks of receiving a transfusion of PRBCs as an intervention. The common finding throughout the literature is that blood transfusion, as an intervention, although necessary and providing therapeutic benefit to most patients, also exposes that patient to a potential increased risk of morbidity and mortality, which is already increased during the critical illness phase of their hospitalization. The systematic review of the literature was limited to studies from 2008 to 2016. Therefore, it is reasonable to conclude that the evidence supported in this systematic review reflects current practice related to single-unit transfusion of PRBCs and patient outcomes for critically ill hospitalized patients who receive this intervention.

Strengths and Limitations of the Systematic Review

The PRISMA guideline used for the review is an effective strategy to use when evaluating scientific research articles that inform clinical practice.[4] Each article was evaluated against the guidelines as a method to achieve comparability, as well as enhanced interrater reliability, with other published systematic reviews. Applying this methodology assures the clinician that only those published studies that meet inclusion criteria will be used as a basis to inform the scientific and clinical body of knowledge as it relates to RBC transfusion interventions in the critical care setting. It is also relevant that the authors of this systematic review included multiple clinical databases to locate articles that describe the current state of scientific study related to this intervention. The systematic review was inclusive of multiple patient conditions and diagnoses, across the entire span of age, and who required intensive or critical care services.

Limitations of this systematic review should also be considered when applying these findings to clinical practice. The use of the RCT study design, considered by most scientific and clinical scholars to be the gold standard of research to inform clinical practice, was limited to 1 study. A variety of other study designs were used and each had some inherent weakness that limited its applicability to clinical practice. Other factors that may limit applicability to practice is that subjects from all age groups were included. The purpose for doing this was deliberate because it would enhance inclusion and inform clinicians of a greater number of possible complications related to blood infusion as an intervention. Clinicians who focus on a particular age group would, therefore, need to identify those risks commonly associated with their patient population. It is apparent to the authors that additional research, using robust study designs that inform clinical practice about the therapeutic benefits, as well as the risk associated with blood transfusion as an intervention in the critically ill patient, is warranted.

REFERENCES

1. Marik PE, Corwin HL. Efficacy of red blood cell transfusion in the critically ill: a systematic review of the literature. Crit Care Med 2008;36(9):2667–74.
2. Kamran MA, Puri N, Gerber DR. Anemia and blood transfusions in critically ill patients. J Blood Transfus 2012;2012:629204.
3. Patel MS, Carson JL. Anemia in the preoperative patient. Med Clin North Am 2009;93(5):1095–104.
4. Liberati A, Altman DG, Tetzlaff J, et al. The PRISMA statement for reporting systematic reviews and meta-analyses of studies that evaluate healthcare interventions: explanation and elaboration. BMJ 2009;339:b2700.
5. Higgins JPT, Green S, editors. Cochrane handbook for systematic reviews of interventions, version 5.1.0 [updated March 2011]. The Cochrane Collaboration, 2011. Available at: www.handbook.cochrane.org.
6. Berger MD, Gerber B, Arn K, et al. Significant reduction of red blood cell transfusion requirements by changing from a double-unit to a single-unit transfusion policy in patients receiving intensive chemotherapy or stem cell transplantation. Hematologica 2012;97(1):116–22.
7. Hajjar LA, Vincent JL, Galas FR, et al. Transfusion requirements after cardiac surgery: the TRACS randomized controlled trial. JAMA 2010;304(1):1559–67.
8. Szpila BE, Ozrazgat-Baslanti T, Zhang J, et al. Successful implementation of a packed red blood cell and fresh frozen plasma transfusion protocol in the surgical intensive care unit. PLoS One 2015;10(5):e0126895.
9. Toy P, Bacchetti P, Grimes B, et al. Recipient clinical risk factors predominate in possible transfusion-related acute lung injury. Transfusion 2015;55(5):947–52.
10. Dos Santos A, Sousa AG, Piotto R, et al. Mortality risk is dose-dependent on the number of packed red blood cell transfused after coronary artery bypass graft. Rev Braz Cir Cardiovasc 2013;28(4):509–17.
11. Rubinstein C, Davenport D, Dunnagan R, et al. Intraoperative blood transfusion of one or two units of packed red blood cells is associated with a fivefold risk of stroke in patients undergoing elective carotid endarterectomy. J Vasc Surg 2013;57(2):53S–7S.
12. Whitlock E, Kim H, Auerbach A. Harms associated with single unit perioperative transfusion: retrospective population based analysis. BMJ 2015;350:h3037.
13. Christou G, Abou-Nassar K, Li Y, et al. A pilot prospective study of the vascular repair response following red cell transfusion in critically ill patients. Transfus Med 2013;23(2):94–9.
14. Kumar R, Gupta M, Gupta V, et al. Acute transfusion reactions (ATRs) in intensive care unit (ICU): a retrospective study. J Clin Diagn Res 2014;8(2):127–9.
15. Zalpuri S, Middelburg R, Schonewille H, et al. Intensive red blood cell transfusions and risk of alloimmunization. Transfusion 2014;54(2):278–84.
16. Shehata N, Forster A, Lawrence N, et al. Transfusion patterns in all patients admitted to the intensive care unit and in those who die in hospital: a descriptive analysis. PLos One 2015;10(9):1–12.

Collaborative Strategies for Management of Obstetric Hemorrhage

Betsy Babb Kennedy, PhD, RN, CNE[a],*,
Suzanne McMurtry Baird, DNP, RN[b,c,1]

KEYWORDS

- Obstetric hemorrhage • Transfusion • Hypovolemic shock • Maternal mortality
- Postpartum hemorrhage

KEY POINTS

- Obstetric hemorrhage is a leading preventable cause of perinatal morbidity and mortality requiring a rapid, coordinated, multidisciplinary response to management to promote optimal outcomes.
- Although blood loss is anticipated at birth, early recognition of excessive blood loss and initiation of pharmacotherapy, medical, and surgical interventions offer progressive management options.
- Goals of management include recognition and management of bleeding, maintaining tissue oxygenation and perfusion, and ongoing monitoring for coagulopathies and complications.

Hemorrhage remains the primary cause of maternal mortality worldwide and the sixth leading cause of death in the United States.[1] Postpartum hemorrhage is the number 1 cause of severe morbidity during hospitalization for birth, despite state and national initiatives.[2] In addition, studies show that more than 90% of maternal deaths related to obstetric hemorrhage are preventable.[1,3,4] The purpose of this article is to review relevant physiologic changes of pregnancy that may have an impact on hemorrhage management, summarize causes of obstetric hemorrhage, and describe collaborative approaches for management of hemorrhage in this unique population.

Disclosure Statement: The authors have nothing to disclose.
[a] Vanderbilt University School of Nursing, 204 Godchaux Hall, 461 21st Avenue South, Nashville, TN 37240, USA; [b] Clinical Concepts in Obstetrics, Inc, Nashville, TN, USA; [c] Labor and Delivery, Vanderbilt University Medical Center, Vanderbilt University School of Nursing, Nashville, TN, USA
[1] Present address: 1180 Manley Lane, Brentwood, TN 37027.
* Corresponding author.
E-mail address: betsy.kennedy@vanderbilt.edu

Crit Care Nurs Clin N Am 29 (2017) 315–330
http://dx.doi.org/10.1016/j.cnc.2017.04.004
0899-5885/17/© 2017 Elsevier Inc. All rights reserved.

CAUSES OF OBSTETRIC HEMORRHAGE

The exact incidence of obstetric hemorrhage is unknown, but risk is present during every pregnancy. In the United States, the incidence of obstetric hemorrhage is 2.9% of all births. The incidence of hemorrhage requiring transfusion has increased by 114%.[2] Although definitions vary, there are some common themes. Obstetric hemorrhage can be viewed as cumulative estimated blood loss of greater than 1000 mL for either vaginal or cesarean birth, associated with signs and symptoms of hypovolemia,[5] but providers should escalate observation and prepare for rapid intervention if blood loss is more than 500 mL to 1000 mL without symptoms. Diagnosis can be problematic due to the typically subjective and inaccurate nature of determining blood loss. Regardless of diagnosis, the following should be considered clinical triggers for heightened observation and action[6]:

1. Heart rate greater than or equal to 110 beats per minute
2. Blood pressure less than or equal to 85/45 mm Hg (>15% drop)
3. Oxygen saturation less than 95%

Causes of obstetric hemorrhage are varied, with the potential for bleeding complications at every stage of pregnancy. Numerous factors associated with hemorrhage in pregnancy, such as body mass index, length of labor, and factors associated with overdistention of the uterus, such as multiple gestation, polyhydramnios, and fetal macrosomia influence risk. Risk assessment is not static, performed only on admission. Risk status for obstetric hemorrhage can change significantly and rapidly, and modifications in the plan of care may be warranted based on ongoing risk assessment. Causes of obstetric hemorrhage relative to timing and risk are presented in **Table 1**. Antepartum and intrapartum hemorrhage is usually associated with abnormal placentation, uterine rupture, or placental abruption. Hemorrhage during the third stage of labor, the first 2 hours of the postpartum period, is the most common time for obstetric hemorrhage to occur. Related postpartum causes can be easily remembered in this manner: tone (70%), trauma (20%), tissue (10%), and thrombin (<1%).[7]

HEMOSTATIC/HEMATOLOGIC ADAPTATIONS OF PREGNANCY

Profound, protective hemodynamic and hematologic changes occur during pregnancy to provide reserve for anticipated blood loss during childbirth. These changes can alter the expected and clinically observed signs of compromise in a hemorrhaging obstetric patient. During pregnancy, blood volume increases by 1600 mL above nonpregnant values.[8] Plasma volume increases 10% to 15% at 6 weeks' to 12 weeks' gestation and plateaus at 40% to 45% at approximately 30 weeks' to 34 weeks' gestation. Later in pregnancy, red blood cell mass increases by 30% to support higher metabolic requirements for oxygen.[9] Hypervolemia in pregnancy further increases with the number of fetuses.[8] Increased blood volume is responsible for an increase in maternal cardiac output of 40% to 50% (6–10 L/min at rest in term gestation). Hormonal changes mediate a decrease in peripheral vascular resistance. Alterations in coagulation factors and the fibrinolytic cascade result in a hypercoagulable state.[10] Thus the mother is prepared with compensatory responses for significant blood loss at birth. Protective physiologic adaptations also result, however, in a mother's ability to experience significant blood loss before tachycardia and hypotension develop. In pregnant women, hypotension and tachycardia are late signs that manifest after blood loss is greater than 15% of circulating blood volume.[11] Physiologic adaptions of the hematologic and hemostatic systems are summarized in **Table 2**.

Table 1
Causes and risk assessments for obstetric hemorrhage

Risk Status	Low	Moderate	High
Prenatal/ antepartum	• Abortion • Ectopic pregnancy • No previous uterine incision or surgery • Singleton pregnancy • ≤4 previous vaginal births • No known bleeding disorders • No previous history of postpartum hemorrhage • Prolonged oxytocin use during labor • Magnesium sulfate administration	• Prior cesarean birth(s) of uterine surgery • Multiple gestation • >4 previous vaginal births • Chorioamnionitis • Previous history of postpartum hemorrhage • Large uterine fibroids	• Placenta previa, low-lying placenta • Suspected morbidly adherent placenta (placenta accreta, placenta percreta, placenta increta) • Hematocrit <30% AND other risk factor • Platelet <100,000 µg/L • Active bleeding on admission
Intrapartum/ postpartum		• Chorioamnionitis • Prolonged oxytocin administration (>24 h) • Prolonged second stage • Magnesium sulfate administration	• Active bleeding on admission

Data from Refs.[14,42,43]

Table 2
Hematologic and hemostatic adaptations of pregnancy

Alterations	Results
↑ Blood volume to 6–7 L ↑ Plasma volume 40% ↑ Plasma renin activity ↓ Atrial natriuretic peptide levels ↑ Erythropoietin levels ↑ Red blood cell mass ↑ Factors II, VII, VIII, X, XII, XIII ↑ von Willebrand ↑ Fibrinogen ↓ Factors XI, XIII = Factors V, IX = Protein C ↑ Thrombin activatable fibrinolytic inhibitor, plasminogen activator inhibitors (PA-1 and PA-2) ↑ Fibrin D-dimer, fibrin monomers, fibrinopeptides A and B ↑ Plasminogen activator, tissue-type plasminogen activator ↑ RBCs 2,3-bisphosphoglycerate ↑ Neutrophils = Platelet count	• Dilutional anemia • Increased efficiency of clotting • Decreased fibrinolysis • Neutrophilia • Mild thrombocytopenia • Decreased oxygen affinity for maternal RBCs

Abbreviations: =, no change in pregnancy; RBC, red blood cell.

OBSTETRIC HEMORRHAGE AND HYPOVOLEMIC SHOCK

If hemorrhage progresses beyond anticipated blood loss for birth, hypovolemic shock can result. Hypovolemic shock occurs when circulating blood volume is decreased by 25% or more and results in insufficient tissue oxygenation. The subsequent release of epinephrine and norepinephrine results in vasoconstriction of both peripheral and central blood vessels. Vasoconstriction in the capillary beds and autotransfusion to the central circulation cause a temporary increase in circulating blood volume. Catecholamine release also increases heart rate, vascular tone, and myocardial contractility in a compensatory response to loss of significant blood volume. Circulating blood volume is redistributed with preferential shunting of blood to the heart, brain, and lungs, away from nonessential organ systems, including the kidneys and uterus. In the absence of circulating volume restoration, compensatory mechanisms fail, resulting in inadequate perfusion, tissue hypoxia, metabolic acidosis, end organ dysfunction, and, ultimately, maternal death. Maternal hemorrhage is sometimes classified by volume of blood loss[12]:

- Class I – 1000 mL
- Class II – 1500 mL
- Class III – 2000 mL
- Class IV – greater than 2500 mL

Maternal symptoms become more prominent as the volume of blood loss increases. If hemorrhage occurs in the antepartum or intrapartum periods, significant disruptions to uterine and placental blood flow can occur. The fetus is at significant risk for progressive physiologic compromise due to decreased oxygen delivery if adequate volume is not restored. Evidence suggestive of fetal compromise in the presence of maternal hemorrhage includes fetal tachycardia, absent fetal heart rate variability, late decelerations, and fetal bradycardia. The risks to both mother and fetus are directly related to both the amount and duration of maternal hemorrhage.

COMMON CARE ISSUES

Many factors can contribute to poor perinatal outcomes with obstetric hemorrhage. Prevention of severe hemorrhage with early recognition and intervention is critical to outcomes. Common areas of concern include

- Failure to accurately estimate and/or measure blood loss and identify hemorrhage
- Failure to monitor based on risk status
- Failure to recognize trends in maternal compromise and communicate assessment findings
- Underestimation of adequate volume required for resuscitation in the presence of hypovolemic shock
- Delay in surgical intervention when manipulation and medication strategies are ineffective at controlling hemorrhage

Health care teams should be knowledgeable of risk and be prepared to respond rapidly with treatment. Management of hemorrhage is framed by goals for treatment, a progression of evidence-based interventions, and strategies to avoid common errors and delays.

GENERAL MANAGEMENT OF OBSTETRIC HEMORRHAGE

Caring for a pregnant woman with a hemorrhage presents unique challenges and requires a multidisciplinary approach to management to optimize maternal and fetal outcomes. Interventions range from simple to complex but must be initiated rapidly in emergent situations. There are 3 overarching goals for treatment:

1. Recognize and *MANAGE* the bleeding
2. *MAINTAIN* tissue oxygenation and perfusion
3. *MONITOR* for coagulopathy and compromise.

Management principles based on these goals can be applied in any obstetric hemorrhage situation, with specific medical or surgical strategies as indicated for the cause.

Physical Assessments

In women at risk for or with suspected obstetric hemorrhage, physical assessments provide clues to recognition and parameters for ongoing monitoring of compromise. Increased frequency of ongoing assessments focused on defined physiologic parameters alert the nurse to potential maternal compromise. Once abnormal assessment parameters are evident, early communication and activation of appropriate response team members for management are crucial. Vital signs should be assessed frequently, noting trends upward in maternal heart rate, which may indicate further bleeding, hypovolemia, and acidosis. Respiratory rate rise in hemorrhage as a physiologic response to an increased need for oxygen in the blood. Rapid, shallow respirations, or air hunger, may lead to acidosis. Blood pressure values initially trend upward due to catecholamine release and peripheral vasoconstriction. Hypotension and narrowed pulse pressure (less than 30 mm Hg) values occur with further compromise and impending shock.[13] A woman's vital signs may not trend outside normal values, however, until she has lost approximately one-third of her total blood volume.[14]

Physical assessment parameters that reflect intravascular volume depletion and decreased cardiac output are outlined in **Table 3**. Altered mental status, as evidenced by anxiety, restlessness, confusion, and decreased level of consciousness, suggest decreased cerebral perfusion and are considered ominous, late signs. Cool, clammy, pale skin; delayed capillary refill; and dry, pale mucous membranes are a result of peripheral vasoconstriction and decreased perfusion. If peripheral vasoconstriction is significant and blood flow to the digits is compromised, pulse oximetry waveforms may become dampened and inhibit the ability to accurately reflect tissue oxygen saturation. Therefore, blood gas analysis may be necessary to follow oxygenation status. Decreased renal perfusion may result in oliguria or anuria. Therefore, hourly assessment of urine output with an indwelling urinary catheter provides data that reflect renal perfusion and, therefore, maternal intravascular volume status and cardiac output.[13]

Critical Care

Invasive hemodynamic monitoring may be indicated depending on the severity of hemorrhage and ability to appropriately resuscitate a woman. Arterial, central venous pressure (CVP) and/or pulmonary artery catheters may be used if additional information is necessary to assess cardiac output and oxygen transport parameters to guide fluid resuscitation efforts. In anticipation of hemorrhage for specific diagnoses, such as anticipated morbidly adherent placenta, placement of invasive hemodynamic lines should be planned in advanced of cesarean birth.[13]

Goal #1: Recognize and Manage Blood Loss

Early recognition, communication, and activation of team members to the bedside are keys to beginning management strategies to control hemorrhage and treat maternal

Table 3
Assessment of hypovolemia

Parameter	Assessment	Rationale
Heart rate	Tachycardia; Heart rate >110 beats per minute and trending upward	Compensatory to maintain cardiac output; caused by catecholamine release; monitor for dysrhythmia
Respiratory rate	Tachypnea; respiratory rate >24 breaths per minute and trending upward	Influence of stress, catecholamine release, hypoxia, and metabolic acidosis due to decreased tissue perfusion
Blood pressure	Initially increased; decreases with lowered cardiac output	Initial increase is compensatory vasoconstriction due to catecholamine release as an attempt to maintain cardiac output; hypotension late sign and associated with shock
Pulse pressure	Narrowing	<30 mm Hg consider shock
SpO_2	Decreased <96%	Inability to monitor as peripheral pulses weaken; increased oxygen utilization
Capillary refill	Prolonged capillary refill >4 s	Decreased arterial width due to decreased intravascular volume
Peripheral pulse quality	Weak, thready progressing to absent	Decreased cardiac preload
Urine output	Oliguria <30 mL urine output for 2 consecutive hours	Decreased kidney perfusion, vasoconstriction, and hypoxia
Skin temperature of extremities	Cool to touch	Peripheral vasoconstriction
Skin color	Pallor	Peripheral vasoconstriction
Mucous membranes	Dry, pale; increased thirst	Decreased intravascular volume
Level of consciousness	Initial anxiety and confusion; may progress to unconscious state	Decreased cerebral perfusion leading to cerebral hypoxia and acidosis; late sign
Cardiac arrest	Pulseless electrical activity	Caused by critical organ failure secondary to blood/fluid loss, hypoxia, dysrhythmia, decreased perfusion

Data from Ruth D, Kennedy B. Acute volume resuscitation following obstetric hemorrhage. J Perinat Neonatal Nurs 2011;25(3);253–60; and Adler AC, Sharma R, Higgins T, et al. Hemodynamic assessment and monitoring in the intensive care unit: an overview. J Anesthes Crit Care Med 2014;1:4–13.

hypovolemia. Responses should be standardized and based on quantified blood loss and/or maternal signs and symptoms of hemorrhage.[15,16] Each member of the hemorrhage response team should be trained to function with specific roles of resuscitation. The Joint Commission on the accreditation of health care organizations; American College of Obstetricians and Gynecologists; Association of Women's Health, Obstetric and Neonatal Nurses; and the National Partnership for Maternal Safety recommend the development and adoption of standardized postpartum hemorrhage protocols to decrease morbidity and mortality.[15–17] Most published protocols provide a staged approach to management based on cumulative blood loss and maternal physiologic response.

Management of obstetric hemorrhage while simultaneously determining the cause of hemorrhage is necessary to improve outcomes for a woman and her fetus.[15] If a woman is still pregnant when a hemorrhage occurs, continuous electronic fetal monitoring should be ongoing to determine fetal status if gestational age is viable and if intervention on behalf of the fetus is planned. Consideration for timing of birth is required with placental conditions, such as abruption, placenta previa, and suspected morbidly adherent placenta. In these scenarios, radiologic studies may be necessary for diagnosis.

Quantitative assessment of blood loss

Accurate assessment of the amount of blood loss is essential in the event of hemorrhage. Visual, estimated blood loss has traditionally been unreliable and inaccurate, potentially delaying timely recognition and management of obstetric hemorrhage.[18,19] Amniotic fluid and irrigation solution can complicate accurate determination of blood loss. Recommended quantification of blood loss (QBL) techniques provide a more objective measurement, improve early recognition, and potentially decrease unnecessary interventions, such as transfusion, surgical intervention, and increased length of stay.[20] Techniques for measuring QBL include weighing blood-saturated items and utilization of collection devices, such as calibrated under-buttocks draping. To quantify blood volume loss by weight, subtract the dry weight of the pads, sponges, or other absorbing materials from the weight of blood-containing materials using a 1-g weight = 1 mL conversion. After vaginal and cesarean birth, prior to delivery of the placenta, providers should stop to assess the collected volume lost and determine a baseline, after which all fluids lost can be considered blood.[20] QBL procedures should be adopted for routine use to standardize processes for quality and safety at all births, rather than implementation after significant blood loss is noticed.[16]

Manipulation and medication

If postpartum hemorrhage occurs, the most common cause is uterine atony (hypotonia). Uterine atony may occur due to overdistention of the uterus with multiple gestations, polyhydramnios, or a macrosomic fetus. In addition, previous postpartum uterine atony, prolonged induction of labor, administration of magnesium sulfate for preeclampsia or preterm labor, intrauterine infection, multiparity, and traumatic birth also increase the risk of postpartum uterine atony. Manipulative measures, including uterine fundal massage and emptying a woman's bladder, are the first 2 steps to improving uterine contractility. Medications are used simultaneously or secondarily to manipulation measures and should be readily available for immediate administration.[15] Oxytocin administration (intravenous [IV] or intramuscular [IM]) is recommended at birth of the fetus or after delivery of the placenta for active management of the third stage of labor to decrease the risk of hemorrhage.[21] In the event of continued uterine atony, several second-line uterotonic agents, such as misoprostol (Cytotec [Pfizer, G.D. Searle, New York, NY]), methylergonovine (Methergine [Novartis AG]), and 15-methyl prostaglandin (Carboprost tromethamine) $F_{2\alpha}$ (Hemabate [Pfizer, New York, NY]), may be required to enhance uterine tone and prevent further blood loss. Off-label administration of recombinant factor VIIa (rFVIIa) may also be considered in severe, uncontrolled obstetric hemorrhage. Ideal obstetric dosing of rFVIIa is not defined, but reported doses are between 40 μg and 90 μg per kilogram.[22] **Table 4** provides information regarding dosing and administration of uterotonic agents. Precise dosing of uterotonic medications, however, are not defined due to lack of controlled comparison trials.

Uterine balloon tamponade

When pharmacologic interventions fail to control postpartum hemorrhage due to uterine atony, placement of a uterine balloon for tamponade is a minimally invasive,

Table 4
Medications

Medication	Dose	Routes	Frequency	Side Effects	Contraindications
Oxytocin (Pitocin)	10–40 U	IV, IM	Continuous IV solution	Nausea and vomiting, water intoxication (high doses)	None
Misoprostol (Cytotec)	400–1000 µg	Oral or rectal	Varies	Nausea, vomiting, diarrhea, fever, chills	None
Methylergonovine (Methergine)	0.2 mg	IM Do not give IV	q 2–4 h for up to 5 doses	Hypertension, nausea and vomiting, myocardial ischemia	Hypertension (chronic or preeclampsia), coronary artery disease
Carboprost tromethamine (Hemabate)	0.25 mg	IM	15–90 min (maximum of 8 doses)	Nausea, vomiting, diarrhea, flushing, fever, vasospasm, bronchospasm	Asthma, cardiac, pulmonary, renal, or hepatic disease

effective adjunct therapy to limit blood loss and gain time for interventions to achieve maternal hemodynamic stability and coagulopath, and possible transfer to another location for care.[5] Balloon tamponade devices can be placed and removed quickly and easily after vaginal or cesarean birth. After examination to eliminate lacerations or retained placental fragments as a cause of postpartum hemorrhage, the tamponade balloon is inserted into the uterus either vaginally or intra-abdominally. The balloon is filled with sterile saline to facilitate compression and slow or stop bleeding within the first 5 minutes to 15 minutes after inflation. The balloon may be left in place for a maximum of 24 hours. Some devices may also include a fluid collection bag to monitor hemostasis and measure any output. An indwelling urinary catheter must be used in tandem if not already placed. Successful use of balloon tamponade may also preserve a woman's reproductive potential for the future.[5]

Antishock garments
Nonpneumatic and pneumatic antishock garments are compression devices used as a temporizing measure to reduce bleeding during hemorrhage by restricting blood flow to the lower body and increasing perfusion to core organs. In the obstetric population, they are most commonly used in areas where resources are scarce but may have usefulness in other settings. If a woman is in a rural or out-of-hospital birth setting, the garments can slow bleeding enough for transport to an inpatient acute care unit. The garments may also slow bleeding in women with continuing hemorrhage who are awaiting arterial embolization in interventional radiology.[23]

Interventional radiology
Interventional radiology and prophylactic arterial placement of balloon catheters for occlusion or embolization of the vessels that perfuse the uterus are also reported as a next-line, more invasive means of controlling hemorrhage, while still preserving future fertility.[24] Bilateral balloon catheters or stents can be placed for occlusion/embolization using angiography. Procedures may also be implemented prior to a planned surgical birth in women with known risks, such as placenta accreta or

placenta percreta. In some cases, a hybrid operating room/interventional radiology suite may be used to expedite treatment and limit transfer of a potentially unstable woman.[25] A multidisciplinary approach and coordination with the interventional radiology team is essential.

Surgical management

Surgical control of hemorrhage should be anticipated in the presence of continued bleeding and/or hemodynamic instability, with early activation of the surgical team for readiness. When manipulation or medication measures to control hemorrhage fail, hesitancy to move to surgical solutions to control bleeding should be avoided.

The type of surgical procedure is dependent on etiology. Common surgical procedures include uterine curettage if retained placental fragments are suspected, placental bed suture, uterine artery ligation, utero-ovarian ligation, repair of uterine rupture, B-Lynch suture for compression of the uterus, laparotomy, and hysterectomy. In addition, transfer to an operative suite may be required for visualization and examination of vaginal or cervical tissue trauma.

Intraoperative cell salvage

Emerging evidence suggests the safe and beneficial use of intraoperative blood salvage (IBS) in the management of obstetric hemorrhage as a surgical management adjunct.[26,27] Theoretical risks of autologous transfusion and IBS in the obstetric population include anaphylactic syndrome of pregnancy due to potential amniotic fluid contamination and the presence of embolic debris and maternal-fetal alloimmunization from the presence of fetal red blood cells. Potential immunization is possible due to the inability of the system to distinguish between maternal and fetal red blood cells, yet the fetal cell transference rate is equivalent to a feto-maternal hemorrhage of any other origin. Therefore, Rho(D) immune globin is administered to Rh-negative women.[27] Anaphylactic syndrome of pregnancy is no longer recognized as an embolic process, so although it may reduce the amount of amniotic fluid collected, there is no evidence to support use of a 2-suction IBS system to prevent the risk of amniotic fluid embolism. A leukocyte depletion filter can also maximize removal of amniotic fluid matter prior to reinfusion.[27] Autologous transfusion may be useful in care of women who decline blood, and consent should be obtained after consultation.[28] IBS-transfused red blood cells do not contain clotting factors, and women experiencing significant hemorrhage and coagulopathy risks require administration of clotting factors and platelets.[28] Considerations for use of IBS include rare maternal blood type or the presence of rare antibodies and availability of equipment and knowledgeable personnel.[29] The decision to have IBS reinfusion equipment available should be based on maternal risk for severe morbidity or mortality with active bleeding.

Acute normovolemic reinfusion

Another transfusion practice alternative when significant bleeding is anticipated, such as in diagnosis of morbidly adherent placenta, is acute normovolemic reinfusion (ANH). ANH involves removal of whole blood and replacement with crystalloid or colloid to maintain intravascular volume during surgery and prior to blood loss. The blood that has been removed is spun down and held in reserve, and then the woman's own packed red blood cells (PRBCs) can be reinfused when indicated.[30] Efficacy in pregnancy is unknown, and safe parameters for hemodilution are not defined.[30] Cell salvage and ANH may be key considerations when an at-risk woman refuses allogenic blood products.

Goal #2: Maintain Perfusion and Oxygenation

Continued significant bleeding can result in hypovolemic shock and decreased circulating blood volume and cardiac output, leading to inadequate tissue perfusion and oxygenation. Compensatory vasoconstrictive responses to hypovolemia can result in tissue hypoxia, metabolic acidosis, and end-organ dysfunction, contributing to significant risk for maternal morbidity and mortality.[31] Hypovolemic shock and disseminated intravascular coagulopathy from hemorrhage are life-threatening complications requiring aggressive management and replacement of intravascular volume to restore cardiac output and oxygen transport.

Oxygenation

Oxygen is administered to maximize available oxygen content with continuous monitoring of oxygen saturation as measured by pulse oximetry (Spo_2) trends. Oxygen administration delays the onset of maternal tissue hypoxia, and, if a woman is still pregnant, the partial pressure of oxygen increases in the maternal circulation, allowing increased availability of oxygen to the fetus.[31] When noting trends to abnormal assessment parameters, oxygen is initiated via non-rebreather facemask at a flow rate of 10 L/min to 12 L/min.

Volume replacement

Prior to central access, peripheral IV access should be accomplished using a large-gauge catheter to increase flow rate. Multiple peripheral IV access lines, depending on severity of hemorrhage, should be considered. Nontunneled central line access allows for additional access infusion ports for large quantities of crystalloids and blood products during an acute hemorrhage and evaluation of right preload (CVP). Because isolated CVP pressures may not accurately reflect left-side heart pressures, management of hemorrhage to adjust preload values should be based on other assessment information and/or trends in CVP data. The preferred central line insertion site during pregnancy is the internal jugular vein due to anatomic changes in pregnancy and risk for pneumothorax.[32]

Initial fluid resuscitation with isotonic crystalloid solutions, lactated Ringer solution, and/or 0.9% sodium chloride meets immediate needs for support, resuscitation, and perfusion. Large-bore IV catheters allow for rapid and aggressive volume expansion. Crystalloids have many advantages, including replenishment of intracellular water and electrolytes, rapid expansion of intravascular volume, low cost, and availability of use. Solutions containing dextrose are avoided for bolus to prevent hyperglycemia in the mother and fetus. Colloid solutions may be used if rapid intravascular volume expansion is required, but there is no evidence for improved outcomes with their use.

Volume replacement is essential, but current evidence supports earlier administration of blood products along with volume. Infusion of large quantities of crystalloid solutions may result in a dilution of plasma proteins, risk for "dilutional coagulopathy", decreased colloid oncotic pressure, increased risk for third spacing of fluid, pulmonary, cerebral and cardiac edema, worsened hemodynamics, and acute kidney injury.[33] In addition, hemorrhage may also be worsened due to increased intravascular hydrostatic pressures resulting in dislodgement of endothelial injury site clots.[22]

Blood component therapy

Intravascular volume resuscitation with crystalloids alone is not sufficient for treatment of severe hemorrhage, because oxygen-carrying capacity must also be improved with red blood cell transfusion. Early identification of fibrinolysis and clotting factor replacement with fresh frozen plasma, cryoprecipitate, and platelets are critical components of hemostatic resuscitation. Alternative blood products and designated volume resuscitation equipment, such as a rapid infuser and cell saver, should be available.

Massive transfusion protocol

Due to the risk of rapid deterioration in maternal and fetal status in the presence of uncontrolled hemorrhage, hospitals must be prepared with a coordinated and practiced massive transfusion protocol (MTP). MTPs are now common and initiated when hemorrhage is expected to be massive (anticipated need to replace 50% or more of blood volume within 2 hours), bleeding continues after the transfusion of 4 U of packed red blood cells within a short period of time (1–2 hours), or systolic blood pressure is less than 90 mm Hg and heart rate above 120 beats per minute in the presence of uncontrolled bleeding.[33–35] If hemorrhage is anticipated, with a diagnosis of suspected morbidly adherent placenta, for example, the MTP may be activated with blood components available in the operative suite prior to surgical birth.[13] An MTP provides guidance on transfusion of packed red blood cells, plasma, platelets, and cryoprecipitate in specific ratios to minimize the effects of dilutional coagulopathy and hypovolemia and allows for earlier administration of blood products in the resuscitation process.[33] Until type-specific blood products are available, emergency release of O-negative PRBCs should be used to prevent a delay in immediate hemorrhage management. Based on risk status (refer to **Table 2**), blood compatibility testing is done on admission.[36]

- Low risk – type and hold
- Moderate risk – type and screen; or, if 2 or more factors are present – type and crossmatch
- High risk – type and crossmatch

The MTP continues in sequence and reactivation until hemostasis occurs in the absence of ongoing hemorrhage. System and process considerations in activation of an MTP include how to activate an MTP, how blood is brought to the patient location, how additional blood products are obtained, and mechanisms for obtaining serial laboratory tests and results with each round of MTP to evaluate transfusion goals.[5] Typical blood component products used in treatment of hemorrhage are described in **Table 5**. Although there is currently limited evidence for use in obstetrics, tranexamic acid (1 g IV over 10 minutes) has also be used for prophylaxis of peripartum bleeding to reduce blood loss and limit the amount of transfusion products.[33] It is not widely available and is not yet universally recommended for use in obstetrics, although it is potentially a safe an effective treatment of obstetric hemorrhage.[33] rFVIIa is typically included as a part of MTP as a second-line treatment after major sources of bleeding have been controlled; however, there are significant concerns about potential thromboembolic events.[33] Laboratory values should be monitored between coolers of blood during an MTP. Initial hematocrit and hemoglobin values immediately after an acute hemorrhage inaccurately reflect the amount of blood loss because plasma and red blood cells are depleted at the same time, requiring at least 2 hours for equilibration. Therefore, initial laboratory values allow for trending in data and results should not be used to determine the need for activation or continuation of the protocol.[33]

Other considerations

The Kleihauer-Betke test is used to detect the presence of fetal cells in maternal circulation occurring as a result of an obstetric event, such as significant hemorrhage.

In Rh-negative women who deliver an Rh-positive fetus, fetomaternal hemorrhage can cause alloimmunization and the possibility of hemolytic disease of the fetus or

Table 5
Blood component therapy

Product	Contents	Effect
PRBCs	Red blood cells, white blood cells, plasma	Increases hematocrit 3% points per unit Increases hemoglobin by 1 g/dL per unit Increases oxygen-carrying capacity Increases preload Increases colloid oncotic pressure
Platelets	Platelets, red blood cells, white blood cells, plasma	Increases platelet count 5000–10,000/mm^3 per unit Enhances clotting capability
Fresh frozen plasma	Fibrinogen, antithrombin III, factors V and VIII	Increases fibrinogen by 10 mg/dL per unit Increases ability to form fibrin clot Increases preload
Cryoprecipitate	Fibrinogen; factors V, VIII, XIII; von Willebrand factor	Increases fibrinogen by 10–15 mg/dL per unit Treatment of von Willebrand disease
Recombinant human coagulation factor VIIa	Off-label adjunct therapy	Decreases bleeding in 85% of cases 90 µg/kg given IV over 3–5 min; repeated in 20 min

newborn in future pregnancies. A prophylactic dose of anti-D immunoglobin can be administered to these women for prevention.

Goal #3: Monitor for Coagulopathy and Complications

Ongoing monitoring of maternal and fetal status is essential to prevent further compromise leading to multisystem organ failure and to assess for improvement of status after interventions. Hemorrhage creates hemostatic imbalances as a result of consumptive or dilutional factors, further increasing the risk of morbidity and mortality associated with hemorrhage. Therefore, effective management is dependent on appropriate monitoring. Adding complexity to the management approach are the normal hemostatic alterations of pregnancy, establishment of reference ranges for pregnancy and transfusion triggers, and the length of turnaround time for standard laboratory testing. Laboratory values for pregnancy are not differentiated in laboratory ranges.

Coagulopathies

Diagnosis of coagulopathies in the obstetric population can be a challenge the normal hemostatic changes, such as elevated fibrinogen levels and fibrinogen-fibrin degradation products.[37] Obstetric hemorrhage is one of the most common conditions resulting in consumptive coagulopathy from the dilutional effect of massive transfusion without replacement of clotting factors, yet it can also occur early in massive hemorrhage without another underlying cause.[37] MTPs, described previously, are now used to guide resuscitation and replacement efforts such that dilutional coagulopathy can be addressed and guide earlier transfusion of fresh frozen plasma. Scoring systems for diagnosis of disseminated intravascular coagulopathy have not been shown effective for use in the obstetric population.

Laboratory screening for coagulation status includes platelet count, prothrombin time, activated partial thromboplastin time, and international normalized ratio; however, it may be of limited value during an acute event. D-dimer values in pregnancy fluctuate dramatically and are not reliable for management decision-making. Plasma fibrinogen levels have been noted to decrease early in the course of obstetric hemorrhage; therefore, waiting to transfuse until fibrinogen levels are significantly low can be too late. Because length of time for obtaining laboratory results can contribute to delays in treatment, resulting in increased risk for morbidity and mortality, trending laboratory assessments should be noted and acted on. Point-of-care testing during an acute hemorrhage may be effective to determine management and decrease delays in laboratory evaluation and communication. Point-of-care testing includes thromboelastography (TEG, Haemoscope, Niles, Illinois) and thromboelastometry (ROTEM, Tem International, Munich, Germany). TEG values can provide a complete, rapid, closer to real time assessment of the speed and quality of clot formation, which, in combination with clinical signs and symptoms, allows for a pathophysiologic, logical guide to intervention to improve outcomes.[38,39] TEG can be run on whole blood and provides information on coagulation factors, platelet function, fibrinogen level, and fibrinolysis.[40]

Complications

After an obstetric hemorrhage, it is important for nurses to monitor for signs and symptoms of potential complications of the hemorrhage or resuscitation, such as third spacing of fluid due to endothelial damage and hypovolemia. Combined with the hematologic hypercoagulable changes in pregnancy, severe hemorrhage places women at increased risk of thromboembolic events due to prolonged surgical procedures, inflammation, and immobilization. After hemorrhage stabilization, prophylactic mechanical compression devices and pharmacologic agents should be initiated.[41] Respiratory compromise from noncardiogenic pulmonary edema should be anticipated with a woman remaining intubated until acute respiratory distress syndrome is ruled out and the extravascular volume shifts back into the vessels. In addition, abdominal compartment syndrome may occur, increasing intra-abdominal pressures and decreasing preload values, cardiac output, and perfusion. Diagnostic criteria of abdominal compartment syndrome include a bladder pressure of greater than 20 mm Hg and dysfunction of 1 organ system.[41] Hypothermia may also result from significant hemorrhage and volume replacement, causing further impairment of oxygen delivery to tissues, decreased cardiac output/cardiovascular response, and decreased functioning of coagulation factors and platelets. Fluid and forced air warmers can be used to maintain body temperature.

CONSIDERATIONS FOR OPTIMIZING CARE
Preparation

Because a hemorrhage can occur at any time, on any shift, obstetric and surgical teams should be ready to intervene at all times. Multidisciplinary team training using simulation and use of protocols is part of a comprehensive strategy to safely and adequately address obstetric hemorrhage. Protocols, such as a postpartum hemorrhage protocol, massive transfusion protocol, hemorrhage bundles, and checklists, can guide providers through evidenced-based steps to provide care in an emergent situation to optimize outcomes. A hemorrhage cart with essential supplies, visual cognitive aids, and checklists for infrequently performed procedures should be readily available on all birthing units for readiness in the event of a hemorrhage.[15]

Communication

All providers on a care team should be empowered to speak up about assessment findings to facilitate appropriate treatment. Care culture that inhibits members of the team from communicating effectively may adversely affect patient outcomes.

Situational awareness of the environment, stage of hemorrhage, maternal assessment parameters, management plans, medications, and completed therapies requires ongoing communication to appropriate care providers and team members. In the event a woman does not stabilize with routine protocol implementation, anticipation, communication, and collaboration for transfer to a higher level of care are necessary.

A Family-Centered Approach

Provision of the right care, at the right time, in the right place, and in a safe manner is the hallmark of quality. Family-centered care should not cease in the event of an emergent obstetric hemorrhage. Inclusion of a woman and her family in multidisciplinary rounds and postevent debriefings to allow for questions enhances communication as well as coordination. With an emergent response, there is not always time to adequately prepare a family, but information should be provided as soon as possible, and the woman and family should be included in decision making. A team member or designee can remain with the family for sensitive support and, where appropriate, a family member may remain with the mother during selected procedures. Although controversial, the benefit of family member presence, even during invasive or resuscitative efforts, has an increasing evidence base.[15]

SUMMARY

Successful management of hemorrhage requires knowledge, skills, awareness of risks, accurate measurement of blood loss, early recognition of maternal compromise, readiness of trained response teams, and swift management to correct the cause while appropriately resuscitation measures are implemented. Delays in management increase the likelihood of maternal and fetal compromise and perinatal morbidity and mortality.

REFERENCES

1. Creanga AA, Berg CJ, Syverson C, et al. Pregnancy-related mortality in the United States, 2006-2010. Obstet Gynecol 2015;125(1):5–12.
2. Callaghan WM, Creanga AA, Kuklina EV. Severe maternal morbidity among delivery and postpartum hospitalizations in the United States. Obstet Gynecol 2012; 120(5):1029–36.
3. Clark SL. Strategies for reducing maternal mortality. Semin Perinatol 2012;36(1): 42–7.
4. Bouvier-Colle MH, Ould El Joud D, Varnoux N, et al. Evaluation of the quality of care for severe obstetrical haemorrhage in three French regions. BJOG 2001; 108(9):898–903.
5. American College of Obstetricians and Gynecologists. Postpartum hemorrhage. Washington, DC: American College of Obstetricians and Gynecologists; October 10, 2006 (ACOG practice bulletin; no. 76).
6. Arafeh J, Gregory K, Main E, et al. Definition, early recognition and rapid response using triggers. California maternal quality care collaborative. CMQCC obstetric hemorrhage toolkit 2015; Available at: https://www.cmqcc.org/resources-tool-kits/toolkits/ob-hemorrhage-toolkit.

7. Anderson JM, Etches D. Prevention and management of postpartum hemorrhage. Am Fam Physician 2007;75(6):875–82.
8. Pritchard J. Changes in blood volume in pregnancy and delivery. Anesthesiology 1965;26:393–8.
9. Conrad LB, Groome LJ, Black DR. Management of persistent postpartum hemorrhage caused by inner myometrial lacerations. Obstet Gynecol 2015;126(2):266.
10. Lockwood C. Pregnancy associated changes in the hemostatic system. Clin Obstet Gynecol 2006;49(4):836–49.
11. Padnamanbhan A, Schwartz J, Spitalnik S. Transfusion therapy in postpartum hemorrhage. Semin Perinatol 2009;33(2):124–7.
12. Francois K, Foley M. Antepartum and postpartum hemorrhage. In: Gabbe S, Simpson J, Neibyl J, editors. Obstetrics: normal and problem pregnancies. 6th edition. New York: Churchill Livingstone; 2012. p. 415–44.
13. Baird S, Troiano N, Kennedy B. Morbidly adherent placenta: interprofessional management strategies for the Intrapartum period. JPNN 2016;30(4):319–26.
14. Harvey CJ, Dildy GAD. Obstetric hemorrhage. In: Troiano NH, Chez BF, Harvey CJ, editors. AWHONN: high risk and critical care obstetrics. 3rd edition. Philadelphia: Lippincott Williams & Wilkins; 2013. p. 246–73.
15. Main E, Goffman D, Scavone B, et al. National partnership for maternal safety: consensus bundle on obstetric hemorrhage. Anesth Analg 2015;121(1):142.
16. Association of Women's Health, obstetric and neonatal nurses. AWHONN postpartum hemorrhage project. 2014. Available at: http://www.pphproject.org/resources.asp. Accessed November 20, 2016.
17. The Joint Commission. Sentinel event alert, issue 44: preventing maternal death. Available at: http://www.jointcommission.org/sentinel_event_alert_issue_44_preventing_maternal_death/. Accessed November 20, 2016.
18. Al Kadri H, Anazi B, Tamim H. Visual estimation versus gravimetric measurement of postpartum blood loss: a prospective cohort study. Arch Gynecol Obstet 2011;283(6):1207–13.
19. Patel A, Goudar S, Geller S, et al. Drape estimation vs. visual assessment for estimating postpartum hemorrhage. Intl J Gynaecol Obstet 2006;93(3):220–4.
20. Gabel KT, Weeber TA. Measuring and communicating blood loss during obstetric hemorrhage. J Obstet Gynecol Neonatal Nurs 2012;41(4):551–8.
21. Association of Women's Health, obstetric and neonatal nurses. Oxytocin administration for management of third stage of labor. Practice brief number 2. Available at: http://www.pphproject.org/downloads/awhonn_oxytocin.pdf. Accessed November 20, 2016.
22. Pacheco LD, Saade GR, Constantine MM, et al. The role of massive transfusion protocols in obstetrics. Am J Perinatol 2013;30(1):1–4.
23. Miller S. Antishock garments: non-pneumatic anti shock garment and pneumatic anti-shock garment. California maternal quality care collaborative. CMQCC obstetric hemorrhage toolkit 2015; Available at: https://www.cmqcc.org/resources-tool-kits/toolkits/ob-hemorrhage-toolkit.
24. American College of Obstetricians and Gynecologists. Placenta accreta. Washington, DC: American College of Obstetricians and Gynecologists; 2012 (Reaffirmed 2014). ACOG committee opinion number 529. Available at: http://www.acog.org/-/media/Committee-Opinions/Committee-on-Obstetric-Practice/co529.pdf?dmc=1&ts=20150403T1044594777.
25. Peralta F, Wong C. Interventional radiology in the pregnant patient for obstetric and non-obstetric indications: organizational, anesthetic, and procedural issues. Int Radiol 2013;26(4):450–5.

26. Milne ME, Yazer MH, Waters JH. Red blood cell salvage during obstetric hemorrhage. Obstet Gynecol 2015;125(4):919–23.
27. Peacock L, Clark V, Catling S. Recent developments in the obstetric use of cell salvage. Transfus Altern Transfus Med 2012;12(3–4):66–71.
28. Liumbruno G, Liumbruno C, Rafanelli D. Intraoperative cell salvage in obstetrics: is it a real therapeutic option? Transfusion 2011;51(10):2244–56.
29. Mercier F, Van De Velde M. Major obstetric hemorrhage. Anesthesiol Clin 2008; 26(1):53–66.
30. Freidman A. Obstetric hemorrhage. J Cardio Vasc Anesth 2013;27(24S):S44–8.
31. Ruth D, Kennedy B. Acute volume resuscitation following obstetric hemorrhage. JPNN 2011;25(3):253–60.
32. Troiano NH, Gattapadi S. Invasive hemodynamic and oxygen transport monitoring during pregnancy. In: Troiano NH, Chez BF, Harvey CJ, editors. AWHONN: high risk and critical care obstetrics. 3rd edition. Philadelphia: Lippincott Williams & Wilkins; 2013. p. 31–46.
33. Pacheco L, Saade G, Constantine M, et al. An update on the use of massive transfusion protocols in obstetrics. Am J Obstet Gynecol 2016;214(3):340–4.
34. Holcomb JB, Tilley BC, Baraniuk S, et al. Transfusion of plasma, platelets, and red blood cells in a 1:1:1 vs. a 1:1:2 ratio and mortality in patients with severe trauma: the PROPPR randomized clinical trial. JAMA 2015;313(5):471–82.
35. Ducloy-Bouthors AS, Susen S, Wong CA, et al. Medical advances in the treatment of postpartum hemorrhage. Anesth Analg 2014;119(5):1140–7.
36. Butwick A, Goodnough L. Transfusion and coagulation management in major obstetric hemorrhage. Curr Opin Anaesthesiol 2015;28(3):275–84.
37. Cunningham G, Nelson D. Disseminated intravascular coagulation syndromes in obstetrics. Obstet Gynecol 2015;126(5):999–1011.
38. Solomon C, Collis RE, Collins PW. Haemostatic monitoring during postpartum haemorrhage and implications for management. Br J Anaesth 2012;109(6): 851–63.
39. Carvalho M, Rodrigues A, Gomes M, et al. Interventional algorithms for the control of coagulopathic bleeding in surgical, trauma, and postpartum settings: recommendations from the share network group. Clin Appl Thromb Hemost 2016; 22(2):121–37.
40. Callum J, Rizoli S. Assessment and management of massive bleeding: coagulation assessment, pharmacologic strategies, and transfusion management. Hematology Am Soc Hematol Educ Program 2012;2012:522–8.
41. Saade A, Constantine MM. Obstetric hemorrhage: recent advances. Clin Obstet Gynecol 2014;57(4):791–6.
42. Lyndon A, Miller S, Huwe V, et al. Blood loss: Clinical techniques for ongoing quantitative measurement. California maternal quality care collaborative. CMQCC obstetric hemorrhage toolkit; Available at: https://www.cmqcc.org/resources-tool-kits/toolkits/ob-hemorrhage-toolkit.
43. Schorn MN, Phillippi JC. Volume replacement following severe postpartum hemorrhage. J Midwifery Womens Health 2014;59:336–43.

Balance Between the Proinflammatory and Anti-Inflammatory Immune Responses with Blood Transfusion in Sepsis

CrossMark

Teresa C. Rice, MD[a], Amanda M. Pugh, MD[a],
Charles C. Caldwell, PhD[a], Barbara St. Pierre Schneider, PhD, RN[b],*

KEYWORDS

- Leukocyte reduction • Immunosuppression • Cytokines • Sepsis • Inflammation
- Blood transfusion

KEY POINTS

- Blood transfusion in critically ill patients, including those with sepsis, remains a complex issue due to the prevalence of transfusion and associated consequences in this patient population.
- Nurses and other health care providers must be diligent in recognizing and managing a worsening immune status to reduce morbidity and mortality in persons with sepsis.
- Health care providers should take advantage of flow cytometry to monitor patients' immune status; for example, blood cytokine levels, immune cell enumeration, and activation can play a role in the assessment of the immune status of persons who receive blood transfusions.

INTRODUCTION

In the United States, 13.6 million units of blood are donated and 21 million blood products are transfused annually.[1] For much of the last century, blood transfusion has been viewed as having clinical benefits. More recently, however, allogenic transfusion has come under increased scrutiny. Initially, transfusion-related infections were the major concern. With modern blood banking techniques, the risk of a major infection risk (per unit of blood; eg, human immunodeficiency virus, hepatitis B and C) is low, ranging

[a] Division of Research, Department of Surgery, College of Medicine, University of Cincinnati, Cincinnati, OH 45267, USA; [b] The Tony and Renee Marlon Angel Network Professorship, School of Nursing, University of Nevada, Las Vegas, 4505 South Maryland Parkway, Box 453018, Las Vegas, NV 89154-3018, USA
* Corresponding author.
E-mail address: barbara.stpierreschneider@unlv.edu

Crit Care Nurs Clin N Am 29 (2017) 331–340
http://dx.doi.org/10.1016/j.cnc.2017.04.003
0899-5885/17/© 2017 Elsevier Inc. All rights reserved.

from 1:220,000 to 1:800,000.[2] Issues surrounding blood transfusion are particularly important in the critically ill. Up to 95% of patients admitted to the intensive care unit (ICU) have anemia of critical illness by the third hospital day.[3] Blood product transfusion occurs in nearly 45% of patients in the intensive care setting. In patients with an ICU length-of-stay longer than 1 week, the proportion of patients transfused increases to 85%.[4,5] Recent findings suggest blood transfusion in critically ill patients is associated with worse outcomes, including higher morbidity and mortality. It remains uncertain whether blood transfusion compounds an immunosuppressive environment, such as that observed in sepsis, which is a leading cause of mortality in the ICU.

Sepsis, the systemic inflammatory response syndrome in the setting of a severe infection, is responsible for more than 150,000 deaths in the United States annually.[6-8] This condition is characterized by an early robust inflammatory response with a concomitant state of persistent immunosuppression.[9-11] With improved treatment algorithms, mortality within the first 3 days of sepsis has been reduced. However, more than 70% of deaths in sepsis occur after the early inflammatory response. Deaths during the immunosuppressive phase are typically due to failure to control the primary infection or acquisition of nosocomial infections.[10] In a postmortem study, 80% of subjects had unresolved septic foci at time of death,[12] highlighting the prevalence of an immunosuppressive state and the lack of ability for bacterial clearance.

Although blood transfusions are prevalent among ICU patients, the criteria for optimal management of anemia during sepsis are not clearly defined. Administration of blood products can influence the host immune response during sepsis. Understanding these alterations is critical to improving patient outcomes.[13] This article discusses recent literature on the associated inflammatory responses that occur with blood transfusion and provides an analysis of alterations in key inflammatory pathways in response to transfusion in a sepsis population.

Immunomodulation from Blood Transfusion

The effects of blood transfusion on the immune system involve both augmentation and suppression of the immune response, a condition called transfusion-related immune modulation (TRIM). Clinically, the immunosuppressive effects of allogenic blood transfusion were first recognized in prolonged graft survival in solid organ transplants in humans and animals.[14,15] The immunosuppressive effect of transfusion is further supported by increased rates of tumor recurrence after surgical resection and increased postoperative infection rates.[16,17] Further, allogeneic blood transfusions were used therapeutically to reduce renal allograft rejection before the availability of effective immunosuppressant drugs.[17]

Leukocytes

Leukocytes present in the blood components and the related expansion of class I and class II human leukocyte antigens distributed on leukocytes are thought to mediate TRIM. Potential cells that can play a role during TRIM are summarized in **Table 1**. These mechanisms include suppression of cytotoxic cell and monocyte activity, release of immunosuppressive prostaglandins, inhibition of interleukin-2 (IL-2) production, and increased suppressor T-cell activity.[17-19] Other mechanisms are increased IL-10 and IL-4 secretion.[20,21] In vitro assays have demonstrated decreased IL-2 secretion[22] and modulation of natural killer (NK) cell activity[17,18] and delayed-type hypersensitivity responses.[23] To prevent or abrogate these immunosuppressive effects and mechanisms, autologous blood or leukoreduced allogenic blood can be used.[24,25] This process reduces leukocyte numbers by 3 logs. The goal of leukoreduction is to avoid the accumulation of bioactive substances implicated in TRIM

Table 1
Immune cells

Cell Type	Function
Leukocytes or white blood cells	Cells of the immune system, including neutrophils, lymphocytes, monocytes, basophils, and eosinophils
Myeloid cells	Lineage of cells that produce neutrophils, monocytes, basophils, eosinophils, erythrocytes, and platelets
Dendritic cells	Antigen presenting cells that initiate the adaptive immune response
Monocytes or macrophages	Monocytes are circulating cells that differentiate into macrophages that migrate to peripheral tissues and organs to eliminate potential threatening organisms or cells by phagocytosis
Neutrophils	Phagocytic cells that are part of the innate immune response that contain granules with microbicidal enzymes
Lymphocytes	T and B cells that function as part of the adaptive immune system determining the specificity of immunity
B cells	Lymphocytes responsible for humoral immunity that once activated become antibody-secreting plasma cells
Cytotoxic T cells	CD8 positive T cells that directly mediate pathogen clearance
T helper cells	CD4 positive T cells that produce cytokines that activate B cells, cytotoxic T cells, and macrophages
Th1 cells	Produce IL-2 that stimulates growth of T cells and IFN-γ that activates macrophages
Th2 cells	Produce IL-4 and IL-5 that stimulate growth of B cells and differentiation to plasma cells
Th17 cells	Produce IL-17 that enhances migration of neutrophils in an inflammatory response and stimulates mucosal immunity
Regulatory or suppressor T cells	Inhibit T helper and T cytotoxic cells
Natural killer cells	Function as part of the innate immune system to kill virus-infected cells and produce IFN-γ to activate macrophages

(summarized in **Table 2**), thereby reducing post-transfusion infections, preventing febrile transfusion reactions, and decreasing human leukocyte antigen alloimmunization and platelet refractoriness in the recipient.

Nonpolar lipids and lysophosphatidylcholines

In addition to residual leukocytes, packed red blood cell (pRBC) units also contain nonpolar lipids and proinflammatory lysophosphatidylcholines (lyso-PCs).[25,26] Lyso-PCs can increase NK and T cell activity, act as NK cell chemoattractants, induce dendritic cell maturation, and stimulate the production of proinflammatory cytokines.[25,27–29] Immunosuppressive eicosanoids (prostaglandins and thromboxanes) also accumulate in pRBCs.[30] Altogether, the presence of these substances results in additional immunomodulation in a transfused patient.

Erythrocytes

Erythrocyte storage may contribute to the negative immune modulating consequences of blood transfusion. Transfusion of red blood cells (RBCs) stored for greater than 2 weeks is associated with increased rates of nosocomial infections, multisystem organ failure, and mortality.[31,32] With increased storage time, RBCs undergo alterations in pH, lactate, nitric oxide, adenosine triphosphate (ATP), and 2,3-diphosphoglycerate.[33,34]

Table 2
Regulatory proteins of immune response

Cytokines	Subtype	Function
Interferon (IFN)- γ	—	Produced by T helper cells to activate and enhance elimination of pathogens by macrophages
Interleukins	—	Cytokines that mediate cellular functions of the immune system
	IL-1	Proinflammatory cytokine produced by macrophages and acts on the hypothalamus to induce fever during infection
	IL-2	T cell growth factor produced by T helper cells to activate both regulatory and effector T cells
	IL-4	Produced by T helper cells to cause proliferation of B cells and production of specific antibodies
	IL-6	Proinflammatory cytokine produced by macrophages and induces production of acute phase proteins
	IL-7	Stimulates stem cells to differentiate into T and B cells
	IL-10	Produced by T2 helper cells to inhibit activation of T1 helper cells
	IL-12	Produced by macrophages to increase the number of T1 helper cells
	IL-17	Produced by T17 helper cells stimulating the migration of neutrophils to the site of inflammation
	IL-27	Proinflammatory and anti-inflammatory effects on T helper cells
Tumor necrosis factor-alpha (TNF-α)	—	Proinflammatory cytokine produced by macrophages that activates neutrophils and enhances migration by increasing production of adhesion molecules

These alterations have been associated with adverse processes, including thrombosis, lung injury, and immunomodulation.[35] Stored RBC units have increased levels of IL-1, keratinocyte chemoattractant, macrophage inflammatory protein 1α, and macrophage inflammatory protein 2 as compared with fresh RBCs.[36] In a murine model, Belizaire and colleagues[36] demonstrated that washing aged RBCs reduced proinflammatory cytokine concentrations after storage such that, when transfused, the systemic inflammatory response in the recipient was attenuated. This finding suggests that washing stored RBCs may improve outcomes in critically ill patients requiring transfusion.

Microparticles

Microparticles (MPs) are small vesicles derived from the cell membrane, ranging from 0.3 μM to 1.0 μM that retain the surface markers of the parent cell and can modulate the immune system.[37] MPs are formed from erythrocytes during morphologic transformation over time.[38] They can then exert their biologic effect via receptor interaction with target cells or direct transfer of their contents.[39] In mice, resuscitation with RBC-derived MPs resulted in increased pulmonary congestion, thickening of alveolar walls, and neutrophil recruitment.[40] Further, increased neutrophil priming and activation following administration of RBC-derived MPs was observed.[40] Recent research has demonstrated that acid sphingomyelinase (Asm) activity in RBCs is associated with MP formation and treatment of RBCs with amitriptyline, an Asm inhibitor, inhibited MP formation during RBC storage. This treatment was associated with reduced lung inflammation following blood transfusion in a murine model.[41] Together, these data demonstrate the significant contribution of RBC-derived MPs to immunomodulation after transfusion.

Host Immune Response in Sepsis

Sepsis refers to the systemic inflammatory response that occurs due to severe infection.[42] Traditionally, research was focused on blunting the initial hyperinflammatory cytokine storm. However, most septic deaths occur during the protracted immunosuppressive phase due to unresolved septic foci or acquisition of nosocomial infections from opportunistic pathogens.[12,43,44] Tissue harvested from spleens or lungs of septic patients had significantly reduced cytokine production, increased expression of inhibitory molecule expression, expansion of T regulatory cell, and myeloid-derived suppressor cell populations. These findings highlight the immunosuppressive state that occurs in sepsis. Studies have demonstrated a significant increase in positive blood cultures due to opportunistic bacteria, such as *Pseudomonas*, *Candida*, *Acinetobacter*, and *Enterococcus*, in late stages of sepsis, depicting the severity of the depressed immune response.[44] Although some patients may die during the acute hyperinflammatory phase, new therapies and treatments are also directed toward ameliorating the immunosuppressive phase during sepsis.

Blood Transfusion in Sepsis

Transfusion goals

In the ICU, blood transfusion is prevalent among patients with sepsis. As previously described, blood transfusion has immune modulating effects. Consequently, understanding the goals of transfusion in sepsis and which patients benefit the most from transfusion is of critical importance. The 2012 Surviving Sepsis Campaign guidelines recommend a target hemoglobin concentration of 7 to 9 g/dL.[45] These recommendations are based on the findings of the Transfusion Requirements in Critical Care Trial that demonstrated a hemoglobin of 7 to 9 g/dL was not associated with increased mortality in comparison with a hemoglobin of 10 to 12 g/dL.[46] Despite these recommendations, Reade and colleagues[47] demonstrated that actual clinical practice is variable for blood transfusion in critical care settings. This variability further highlights the need to understand the risks of transfusion in critically ill patients to deliver effective care to patients with sepsis.

Patient mortality

Studies have examined whether blood transfusion increases patient mortality. To discuss this effect, an examination of both the sepsis and nonsepsis critically ill literature is necessary. Of note, blood transfusion itself is a marker for severity of illness, complicating the ability to assess mortality following transfusion. In addition, there is a positive correlation between number of transfusion units and mortality.

Findings that show blood transfusions increase mortality involve hip or cardiac surgery or intensive care following trauma or surgery. In a retrospective review, Hebert and colleagues[48] demonstrated that patient mortality increased with transfusion in comparison with that of without transfusion. However, this increased mortality was reduced with leukoreduction.[48] Furthermore, through an analysis of data from 5 cardiac-surgery randomized controlled trials, Vamvakas and colleagues[19] reported that increased short-term mortality (up to 3 months following transfusion) was observed in patients receiving transfusion. However, others have suggested that there is no difference in mortality in surgical patients.[49] Additional randomized controlled studies are necessary to address the effect of blood transfusions on the mortality of patients with sepsis.

Effect on immune mediators

The literature of the effects of blood transfusion on immune mediators in critical illness in patients covers both animal and human studies. An initial report regarding transfusion in septic rats indicates that blood transfusion exacerbates sepsis-induced immunosuppression.[50] Transfusion during sepsis resulted in the downregulation of blood tumor necrosis factor-alpha (TNF)-α and interferon-gamma (IFN)-γ levels, as well as an impaired cellular immune response through decreased CD4 populations.[51]

Similar immunosuppressive effects have been observed in humans. It was reported that patients receiving blood transfusions had a 70% reduction in IL-2, TNF-α, and IFN-γ.[52] These researchers reported alterations in cytokine profiles and reductions in cytotoxic cells, which will contribute to decreased resistance to bacterial infection. More recently, Torrance and colleagues[53] found that anti-inflammatory mediators, IL-10 and IL-27, which suppress the T helper (Th)17 proinflammatory response, were elevated in critically ill polytrauma subjects receiving an immediate blood transfusion. These initial alterations were observed less than 2 hours following transfusion. Further, they observed a direct correlation between the number of transfused units and IL-10 levels. In contrast, the proinflammatory mediator TNF-α had a less significant increase. Greater reductions in IFN-γ and Th17 transcription factors were also observed. Altogether, these data point to the immunosuppressive nature of the response in critically ill patients.

Infection

The potential for TRIM to aggravate the aberrant immune response in sepsis and increase infectious complications is of significant concern. As previously described, blood transfusion can negatively alter the T and NK cell function, which can result in increased susceptibility to nosocomial infection. This effect is supported by increased rates of bacterial infection following surgery and blood transfusion.[54,55] Further, a multivariate analysis suggests that blood transfusion is an independent risk factor for infection but that the risk is reduced with leukoreduced blood.[55–59] Houbiers and colleagues[60] demonstrated an associated dose response between the number of transfused RBC units and the incidence of postoperative infection, including pneumonia, urinary tract infection, infected hematomas, and septicemia. In 2015, Torrance and colleagues[53] concluded that blood transfusion exacerbates the immunosuppressive response in critically ill polytrauma patients, noting an increased susceptibility to infections that was independent of the injury severity score.

SUMMARY

Blood transfusion in critically ill patients, including those with sepsis, remains a complex issue due to the prevalence of transfusion and associated consequences in this patient population. Through the authors' review of the literature, we conclude that blood product transfusion may exacerbate the initial immunosuppressive response of sepsis. Therefore, nurses and other health care providers must be diligent in recognizing and managing a worsening immune status. For example, monitoring the absolute lymphocyte count may be one simple way to detect a worsening immune status[61] because an absolute lymphocyte count of 0.6 cells per microliter or less at 4 days after a diagnosis of sepsis has been observed to be associated with the occurrence of secondary infections and mortality.[62] Additionally, health care providers should take advantage of flow cytometry to monitor patients' immune status.[13] For example, blood cytokine levels and immune cell enumeration and activation can play a role in the assessment of the immune status of persons who receive blood transfusions.[61] This type of monitoring may be instrumental in reducing morbidity and mortality in persons with sepsis.

REFERENCES

1. American Red Cross. Blood facts and statistics. American Red Cross. Available at: http://www.redcrossblood.org/learn-about-blood/blood-facts-and-statistics. Accessed December 21, 2016.
2. Busch MP, Kleinman SH, Nemo GJ. Current and emerging infectious risks of blood transfusions. JAMA 2003;289(8):959–62.
3. Rodriguez RM, Corwin HL, Gettinger A, et al. Nutritional deficiencies and blunted erythropoietin response as causes of the anemia of critical illness. J Crit Care 2001;16(1):36–41.
4. Corwin HL, Gettinger A, Pearl RG, et al. The CRIT study: anemia and blood transfusion in the critically ill–current clinical practice in the United States. Crit Care Med 2004;32(1):39–52.
5. Vincent JL, Baron JF, Reinhart K, et al. Anemia and blood transfusion in critically ill patients. JAMA 2002;288(12):1499–507.
6. Hall MJ, Williams SN, DeFrances CJ, et al. Inpatient care for septicemia or sepsis: a challenge for patients and hospitals. NCHS Data Brief 2011;62:1–8. Available at: http://www.cdc.gov/nchs/data/databriefs/db62.htm. Accessed December 21, 2016.
7. Centers for Disease Control and Prevention. Sepsis data reports. Center for Disease Control and Prevention; 2016. Available at: https://www.cdc.gov/sepsis/datareports/index.html. Accessed December 21, 2016.
8. Moore JX, Donnelly JP, Griffin R, et al. Defining sepsis mortality clusters in the United States. Crit Care Med 2016;44(7):1380–7.
9. Hotchkiss RS, Monneret G, Payen D. Sepsis-induced immunosuppression: from cellular dysfunctions to immunotherapy. Nat Rev Immunol 2013;13(12):862–74.
10. Hotchkiss RS, Monneret G, Payen D. Immunosuppression in sepsis: a novel understanding of the disorder and a new therapeutic approach. Lancet Infect Dis 2013;13(3):260–8.
11. Hutchins NA, Unsinger J, Hotchkiss RS, et al. The new normal: immunomodulatory agents against sepsis immune suppression. Trends Mol Med 2014;20(4): 224–33.
12. Torgersen C, Moser P, Luckner G, et al. Macroscopic postmortem findings in 235 surgical intensive care patients with sepsis. Anesth Analg 2009;108(6):1841–7.
13. Kuethe JW, Mintz-Cole R, Johnson BL 3rd, et al. Assessing the immune status of critically ill trauma patients by flow cytometry. Nurs Res 2014;63(6):426–34.
14. Alexander JW, Babcock GF, First MR, et al. The induction of immunologic hyporesponsiveness by preoperative donor-specific transfusions and cyclosporine in human cadaveric transplants. A preliminary trial. Transplantation 1992;53(2):423–7. Available at: http://journals.lww.com/transplantjournal/Citation/1992/02010/THE_INDUCTION_OF_IMMUNOLOGIC_HYPRESPONSIVENESS_BY.30.aspx. Accessed December 21, 2016.
15. Salvatierra O Jr, Vincenti F, Amend W, et al. Deliberate donor-specific blood transfusions prior to living related renal transplantation. A new approach. Ann Surg 1980;192(4):543–52.
16. Gianotti L, Pyles T, Alexander JW, et al. Identification of the blood component responsible for increased susceptibility to gut-derived infection. Transfusion 1993;33(6):458–65.

17. Cata JP, Wang H, Gottumukkala V, et al. Inflammatory response, immunosuppression, and cancer recurrence after perioperative blood transfusions. Br J Anaesth 2013;110(5):690–701.

18. Jensen LS, Andersen AJ, Christiansen PM, et al. Postoperative infection and natural killer cell function following blood transfusion in patients undergoing elective colorectal surgery. Br J Surg 1992;79(6):513–6.

19. Vamvakas EC. Possible mechanisms of allogeneic blood transfusion-associated postoperative infection. Transfus Med Rev 2002;16(2):144–60.

20. Kirkley SA, Cowles J, Pellegrini VD, et al. Blood transfusion and total joint replacement surgery: T helper 2 (TH2) cytokine secretion and clinical outcome. Transfus Med 1998;8(3):195–204.

21. Karam O, Tucci M, Toledano BJ, et al. Length of storage and in vitro immunomodulation induced by prestorage leukoreduced red blood cells. Transfusion 2009; 49(11):2326–34.

22. Vlaar AP, Hofstra JJ, Kulik W, et al. Supernatant of stored platelets causes lung inflammation and coagulopathy in a novel in vivo transfusion model. Blood 2010;116(8):1360–8.

23. Baumgartner JM, Nydam TL, Clarke JH, et al. Red blood cell supernatant potentiates LPS-induced proinflammatory cytokine response from peripheral blood mononuclear cells. J Interferon Cytokine Res 2009;29(6):333–8.

24. Cardo LJ, Wilder D, Salata J. Neutrophil priming, caused by cell membranes and microvesicles in packed red blood cell units, is abrogated by leukocyte depletion at collection. Transfus Apher Sci 2008;38(2):117–25.

25. Fox LM, Cox DG, Lockridge JL, et al. Recognition of lyso-phospholipids by human natural killer T lymphocytes. PLoS Biol 2009;7(10):e1000228.

26. Silliman CC, Clay KL, Thurman GW, et al. Partial characterization of lipids that develop during the routine storage of blood and prime the neutrophil NADPH oxidase. J Lab Clin Med 1994;124(5):684–94. Available at: https://www.ncbi.nlm. nih.gov/pubmed/7964126. Accessed December 21, 2016.

27. Coutant F, Perrin-Cocon L, Agaugue S, et al. Mature dendritic cell generation promoted by lysophosphatidylcholine. J Immunol 2002;169(4):1688–95.

28. Jin Y, Damaj BB, Maghazachi AA. Human resting CD16-, CD16+ and IL-2-, IL-12-, IL-15- or IFN-alpha-activated natural killer cells differentially respond to sphingosylphosphorylcholine, lysophosphatidylcholine and platelet-activating factor. Eur J Immunol 2005;35(9):2699–708.

29. Olofsson KE, Andersson L, Nilsson J, et al. Nanomolar concentrations of lysophosphatidylcholine recruit monocytes and induce pro-inflammatory cytokine production in macrophages. Biochem Biophys Res Commun 2008;370(2): 348–52.

30. Jacobi KE, Wanke C, Jacobi A, et al. Determination of eicosanoid and cytokine production in salvaged blood, stored red blood cell concentrates, and whole blood. J Clin Anesth 2000;12(2):94–9.

31. Offner PJ, Moore EE, Biffl WL, et al. Increased rate of infection associated with transfusion of old blood after severe injury. Arch Surg 2002;137(6):711–6 [discussion: 716–7].

32. Zallen G, Offner PJ, Moore EE, et al. Age of transfused blood is an independent risk factor for postinjury multiple organ failure. Am J Surg 1999;178(6):570–2.

33. Makley AT, Goodman MD, Friend LA, et al. Murine blood banking: characterization and comparisons to human blood. Shock 2010;34(1):40–5.

34. Sparrow RL. Red blood cell storage and transfusion-related immunomodulation. Blood Transfus 2010;8(Suppl 3):s26–30.

35. Silliman CC, Moore EE, Kelher MR, et al. Identification of lipids that accumulate during the routine storage of prestorage leukoreduced red blood cells and cause acute lung injury. Transfusion 2011;51(12):2549–54.

36. Belizaire RM, Makley AT, Campion EM, et al. Resuscitation with washed aged packed red blood cell units decreases the proinflammatory response in mice after hemorrhage. J Trauma Acute Care Surg 2012;73(2 suppl 1):S128–33.

37. Prakash PS, Caldwell CC, Lentsch AB, et al. Human microparticles generated during sepsis in patients with critical illness are neutrophil-derived and modulate the immune response. J Trauma Acute Care Surg 2012;73(2):401–6 [discussion: 406–7].

38. Gyorgy B, Szabo TG, Pasztoi M, et al. Membrane vesicles, current state-of-the-art: emerging role of extracellular vesicles. Cell Mol Life Sci 2011;68(16):2667–88.

39. Mause SF, Weber C. Microparticles: protagonists of a novel communication network for intercellular information exchange. Circ Res 2010;107(9):1047–57.

40. Belizaire RM, Prakash PS, Richter JR, et al. Microparticles from stored red blood cells activate neutrophils and cause lung injury after hemorrhage and resuscitation. J Am Coll Surg 2012;214(4):648–55 [discussion: 656–7].

41. Hoehn RS, Jernigan PL, Japtok L, et al. Acid sphingomyelinase inhibition in stored erythrocytes reduces transfusion-associated lung inflammation. Ann Surg 2016. http://dx.doi.org/10.1097/SLA.0000000000001648.

42. Vincent JL, Opal SM, Marshall JC, et al. Sepsis definitions: time for change. Lancet 2013;381(9868):774–5.

43. Boomer JS, To K, Chang KC, et al. Immunosuppression in patients who die of sepsis and multiple organ failure. JAMA 2011;306(23):2594–605.

44. Otto GP, Sossdorf M, Claus RA, et al. The late phase of sepsis is characterized by an increased microbiological burden and death rate. Crit Care 2011;15(4):R183.

45. Dellinger RP, Levy MM, Rhodes A, et al. Surviving sepsis campaign: international guidelines for management of severe sepsis and septic shock: 2012. Crit Care Med 2013;41(2):580–637.

46. Hebert PC, Wells G, Blajchman MA, et al. A multicenter, randomized, controlled clinical trial of transfusion requirements in critical care. Transfusion requirements in critical care investigators, Canadian critical care trials group. N Engl J Med 1999;340(6):409–17.

47. Reade MC, Huang DT, Bell D, et al. Variability in management of early severe sepsis. Emerg Med J 2010;27(2):110–5.

48. Hebert PC, Fergusson D, Blajchman MA, et al. Clinical outcomes following institution of the Canadian universal leukoreduction program for red blood cell transfusions. JAMA 2003;289(15):1941–9.

49. Baron JF, Gourdin M, Bertrand M, et al. The effect of universal leukodepletion of packed red blood cells on postoperative infections in high-risk patients undergoing abdominal aortic surgery. Anesth Analg 2002;94(3):529–37. Table of contents.

50. Salinas JC, Cabezali R, Torcal J, et al. Immune response and cytokines in septic rats undergoing blood transfusion. J Surg Res 1998;80(2):295–9.

51. Sousa R, Salinas JC, Navarro M, et al. Autologous blood transfusion as an immunomodulator in experimental sepsis. Int J Surg Investig 2000;1(5):365–71. Available at: https://www.ncbi.nlm.nih.gov/labs/journals/int-j-surg-investig/. Accessed December 21, 2016.

52. Kalechman Y, Gafter U, Sobelman D, et al. The effect of a single whole-blood transfusion on cytokine secretion. J Clin Immunol 1990;10(2):99–105.

53. Torrance HD, Brohi K, Pearse RM, et al. Association between gene expression biomarkers of immunosuppression and blood transfusion in severely injured polytrauma patients. Ann Surg 2015;261(4):751–9.

54. Tang R, Chen HH, Wang YL, et al. Risk factors for surgical site infection after elective resection of the colon and rectum: a single-center prospective study of 2,809 consecutive patients. Ann Surg 2001;234(2):181–9.

55. Acheson AG, Brookes MJ, Spahn DR. Effects of allogeneic red blood cell transfusions on clinical outcomes in patients undergoing colorectal cancer surgery: a systematic review and meta-analysis. Ann Surg 2012;256(2):235–44.

56. Cervia JS, Wenz B, Ortolano GA. Leukocyte reduction's role in the attenuation of infection risks among transfusion recipients. Clin Infect Dis 2007;45(8):1008–13.

57. Fung MK, Rao N, Rice J, et al. Leukoreduction in the setting of open heart surgery: a prospective cohort-controlled study. Transfusion 2004;44(1):30–5.

58. Sievert A. Leukocyte depletion as a mechanism for reducing neutrophil-mediated ischemic-reperfusion injury during transplantation. J Extra Corpor Technol 2003; 35(1):48–52. Available at: http://amsect.smithbucklin.com/JECT/PDFs/2003_volume35/issue1/ject_2003_v35_n1_sievert_a.pdf. Accessed December 21, 2016.

59. Tartter PI, Mohandas K, Azar P, et al. Randomized trial comparing packed red cell blood transfusion with and without leukocyte depletion for gastrointestinal surgery. Am J Surg 1998;176(5):4626.

60. Houbiers JG, van de Velde CJ, van de Watering LM, et al. Transfusion of red cells is associated with increased incidence of bacterial infection after colorectal surgery: a prospective study. Transfusion 1997;37(2):126–34.

61. Patil NK, Bohannon JK, Sherwood ER. Immunotherapy: a promising approach to reverse sepsis-induced immunosuppression. Pharmacol Res 2016;111:688–702.

62. Drewry AM, Samra N, Skrupky LP, et al. Persistent lymphopenia after diagnosis of sepsis predicts mortality. Shock 2014;42(5):383–91.

Nursing Care of Adult Hematopoietic Stem Cell Transplant Patients and Families in the Intensive Care Unit

An Evidence-based Review

Linda K. Young, PhD, RN, CNE, CFLE[a],*,
Brianne Mansfield, DNP, RN, APRN, NP-C[b], Jared Mandoza, BSN, RN[a]

KEYWORDS

- Hematopoietic stem cell transplant (HSCT) • Bone marrow transplant
- Intensive care unit (ICU) • Nursing care • Adult patients and their families
- ICU staff preparation for care

KEY POINTS

- There is limited evidence available addressing the unique needs and interventions for hematopoietic stem cell transplant (HSCT) patients in the intensive care unit (ICU), their families, and the non-HSCT specialized ICU care providers.
- ICU admission for the HSCT adult patients occurs when patients require a higher level of care than can be provided in a non-ICU environment.
- Identifying the relevant medical and nursing diagnoses on admission to the ICU is key.
- Three major areas of interventions are education, communication, and support for patients, families, and non-HSCT–trained providers in the ICU.

For individuals with a hematologic malignancy, a hematopoietic stem cell transplant (HSCT) can be a lifesaving option. HSCT has replaced the previous terminology of bone marrow transplant to reflect a broader and expanding range of cell sources and collection techniques.[1] HSCT treatment consists of chemotherapy followed by stem cell rescue from an autologous transplant (patient's own cells), an allogeneic transplant (stem cells from a donor), or an umbilical cord blood

Disclosure: There was no funding support for this article. None of the 3 authors has any relationship with a commercial company having a direct financial interest in the subject matter or materials discussed in this article or with a company making a competing product.
[a] Department of Nursing, College of Nursing and Health Sciences, University of Wisconsin-Eau Claire, 105 Garfield Avenue, Eau Claire, WI, 54701, USA; [b] Radiation Oncology, Mayo Clinic, 200 First Street Southwest, Rochester, MN 55905, USA
* Corresponding author.
E-mail address: younglk@uwec.edu

Crit Care Nurs Clin N Am 29 (2017) 341–352
http://dx.doi.org/10.1016/j.cnc.2017.04.009
0899-5885/17/© 2017 Elsevier Inc. All rights reserved.

ccnursing.theclinics.com

transplant. For the purpose of this article, allogeneic and autologous transplant are discussed.

HSCT patients are a growing population. In 2012, an estimated 20,000 people received blood/cell transplant in the United States.[1] Between the years 2008 and 2012, there was an incident rate of 13.2 per 100,000 of the US population for leukemia.[2] The incident rate was 19.2 per 100,000 for non-Hodgkin lymphoma.[3] In 2016, the most common reported[4] diagnoses indicating an HSCT included:

- Acute lymphoblastic leukemia (ALL)
- Acute myelogenous leukemia (AML)
- Chronic lymphocytic leukemia (CLL)
- Chronic myelogenous leukemia (CML)
- Lymphomas (Hodgkin and non-Hodgkin)

The numbers of new cases of leukemia and non-Hodgkin lymphoma in the year 2016 are estimated to be 60,140 and 20,150 respectively.[3] These statistics highlight the relevance of HSCT and the increasing patient population.

Depending on the type of transplant, acute and long-term outcomes may vary. The long-term cause of mortality for autologous transplants remains the primary hematologic disease.[2] For allogeneic transplant patients, specifically those receiving cells from an unrelated donor, the cause of mortality is often infections or organ failure.[2] Although both types of transplant go through similar experiences, more complications can arise during allogeneic transplant. Knowing this, nurses can individualize care for adult HSCT patients and their families and lead collaborative efforts for best practice between the multidisciplinary teams working with each patient. To achieve that goal, nurses need to understand the vulnerabilities of HSCT patients, be aware of what nursing and medical diagnoses are present, and cater to patient and family needs at different care transitions, especially before, during, and after an intensive care unit (ICU) experience.

Each transplant center is uniquely designed and has different infrastructure and available resources. In 2015, there were 108 adult centers offering HSCT programs in the United States.[2] Some HSCT programs operate as an inpatient unit located within a hospital. Others operate as a hybrid between inpatient and outpatient centers. Thus, a variety of practices in caring for and supporting patients through transplant occur because of available resources of infrastructure, personnel, and support.[2] The variability in HSCT centers affects the care that staff are able to provide HSCT patients and families.

Both types of transplants, autologous and allogeneic, have the potential of extending life; however, they both involve intense therapy with potentially life-threatening outcomes. The intensity of transplant creates unique health care needs. Acutely, patients are treated in a dynamic environment that spans outpatient, inpatient, and potential ICUs with a multidisciplinary team caring for them. It can be overwhelming for patients and their families to understand their disease, the HSCT treatment effects, and potential complications. This consideration is especially important during care transitions, because patients are fragile and vulnerable to adverse outcomes. This article addresses the unique needs of adult HSCT patients and their families and nonspecialized health care staff specifically when admitted to an ICU environment.

LITERATURE SEARCH

CINAHL Complete, Medline, Cochrane Library, and Center for International Blood and Marrow Transplant Research (CIBMTR) were the databases and sites searched for this article. Search terms included "hematopoietic stem cell transplantation," "bone marrow transplantation," "intensive care unit (ICU)," "nursing care, adult patients and their families," and "ICU staff preparation for care."

Exclusion criteria included pediatric HSCT patients and articles not in English. Inclusion criteria included autogeneic and allogeneic transplant adult patients. Forty-one articles were retrieved and 36 were used as the foundation for this article.

ADMISSION TO INTENSIVE CARE UNIT
Criteria for Admission

There is a significant number of patients who experience complications severe enough to require ICU care during the transplant experience.[5–7] Compared with a general hospital floor, ICUs offer a higher staff to patient ratio as well as the ability to implement life-sustaining measures when a patient's status is deteriorating. Equipment found in the ICU that is necessary to aggressively monitor or provide support to a patient may include mechanical ventilators, telemetry, arterial lines, Swan-Ganz catheters, and dialysis equipment. ICU admission is indicated when a patient is in need of management of organ failure from complications of the disease or complications of the treatment regimen of the disease.[8] The most common reason reported[5,9–14] for admission to the ICU is respiratory failure, followed by:

- Sepsis/shock
- Neurologic failure
- Acute renal failure
- Acute bleeding
- Infection
- Multiorgan failure
- Cardiac failure
- Metabolic disorders

Average Stay in Intensive Care Unit

There are numerous factors that determine the length of stay for HSCT patients in the ICU. Each patient responds differently to the transplant process as well as to the chemotherapy regimen, leading to a varying amount of time the patients need to be supported in the ICU setting. The average length of stay of adult HSCT patients in the ICU is approximately 8 days, ranging from 4 to 14 days.[5,8,9,11,12] If a patient is admitted to the ICU soon after a transplant it is likely to be because of the neutropenic state of the patient and the side effects of immunosuppressive drugs.[12] The neutropenic state puts patients at risk for infection and organ complications associated with those infections (eg, pneumonia and respiratory failure). Patients admitted later in the transplant process are typically admitted for complications of graft-versus-host disease.[12] Complications of graft-versus-host disease can affect any body system and can be seen acutely in the first 100 days and chronically after the first 100 days posttransplant.

Morbidity

During transplant, patients experience many complications from chemotherapy, prolonged neutropenia, and adverse events from polypharmacy. Some of the morbidities associated with transplant are similar to the reasons for ICU admission. The potential complications reported[15] include:

- Infection
- Bleeding

- Anemia
- Gastrointestinal complications
- Renal toxicity
- Hepatic toxicity
- Bladder toxicity
- Pulmonary toxicity
- Cardiac toxicity
- Skin toxicity
- Failed or delayed engraftment
- Graft-versus-host disease

The morbidity of transplant patients occurs in the acute phase of HSCT as well as the long-term phase. These comorbidities caused by HSCT therapy can mean possible or recurrent hospitalizations and ICU admissions.

Mortality

Patients who require ICU care are at higher risk of mortality during their stay and after discharge. Of those admitted to the ICU posttransplant, the most common cause of death is multisystem organ failure. One study found that all patients admitted to ICU because of multisystem organ failure had died within 12 months.[8] Note that the survival of patients who undergo a hematologic stem cell transplant is not dependent on admission to the ICU but is most dependent on the resolution of the acute symptoms of the disease that resulted in them being admitted to ICU.[8] The total number of deaths from leukemia in 2016 for the United States is estimated to be 24,400 and the total number of deaths from non-Hodgkin lymphoma is estimated to be 20,150.[3] Based on the uniqueness of the pathophysiology of the different disease processes as well as the type of transplant, survival posttransplant varies. This variability is reflected in **Table 1**, which provides percentages of survival probability at 100 days and 1 year posttransplant by diseases and type of transplant.[4]

INTERVENTION RECOMMENDATIONS

Based on the review of literature, education, communication, support, and specific care provide a framework for staff, patient, and family interventions when adult HSCT patients are admitted to the ICU.

STAFF INTERVENTIONS
Education

To improve patient and family outcomes in HSCT, adequate staff education as well as care coordination and communication are necessary between and among health care staff in the HSCT specialty areas and the ICU. First, adequate training during orientation can help prepare nurses and other health care providers for the unique care needs of HSCT patients.[16] Many centers have adopted education programs with didactic topics to cover during orientation or ongoing educational sessions to improve staff education. One study focused on 3 topic areas: HSCT core curriculum, essential RN skills, and HSCT supportive care issues.[17] These programs standardize staff education with staff having reported feeling more confident in taking care of HSCT patients.[17,18] Understanding which medical and nursing diagnoses are present when HSCT patients are admitted to the ICU is key. **Table 2** provides the medical diagnoses and correlating NANDA-I (North American Nursing Diagnosis Association)[19] taxonomy nursing diagnoses for HSCT patients admitted to the ICU.

Table 1
Health Resources and Service Administration United States patient survival report: 2008 to 2012

Diseases Categorized by First Remission/Chronic Phase	100-d Posttransplant Survival Probability Estimate (%)	1-y Posttransplant Survival Probability Estimate (%)
ALL		
Autologous	90.5	—
Allogeneic (related)	93.9	77.3
Allogeneic (unrelated)	89.8	71.0
AML		
Autologous	97.3	75.4
Allogeneic (related)	93.3	72.5
Allogeneic (unrelated)	88.3	64.8
CLL		
Autologous	85.2	89.9
Allogeneic (related)	91.5	76.8
Allogeneic (unrelated)	88.1	66.8
CML		
Autologous	—	—
Allogeneic (related)	96.4	79.2
Allogeneic (unrelated)	87.6	69.0
Hodgkin Lymphoma		
Autologous	98.3	95.4
Allogeneic (related)	—	—
Allogeneic (unrelated)	—	—
Non-Hodgkin Lymphoma		
Autologous	97.4	87.3
Allogeneic (related)	84.0	68.0
Allogeneic (unrelated)	87.5	—

Adapted from Health Resources and Service Administration (HRSA). 2016. Available at: https://www.hrsa.gov/index.html.

Note that several nursing diagnoses relevant to HSCT patients and their families exist beyond those correlated with medical diagnoses. Additional nursing diagnoses reported[1,13,24,26–30] in this population in the ICU include:

- Death anxiety
- Depression
- Fear
- Helplessness
- Sleep deprivation
- Spiritual distress
- Interrupted family processes
- Caregiver role strain
- Ineffective relationship
- Pain
- Fatigue
- Decisional conflict

Table 2
Correlating nursing diagnoses with medical diagnoses in intensive care units

Medical Diagnoses	Correlating Nursing Diagnoses
Respiratory failure	Ineffective airway clearance Risk for aspiration Risk for altered breathing pattern Impaired spontaneous ventilation Risk for dysfunctional ventilator weaning response Risk for impaired oral mucous membranes Impaired verbal communication Anxiety/fear
Sepsis/septic shock	Risk for infection (spread) Hyperthermia Risk for ineffective peripheral tissue perfusion Risk for shock Ineffective tissue perfusion Anxiety
Neurologic failure/ seizure/intracranial bleed	Risk for trauma/suffocation Acute confusion
Acute renal failure	Excess fluid volume Risk for imbalanced nutrition: less than body requirements Risk for disturbed thought processes Risk for infection Ineffective protection Impaired urinary elimination
Acute bleed	Ineffective peripheral tissue/renal/gastrointestinal/cerebral perfusion
Infection	Risk for infection Hyperthermia Risk for shock Ineffective protection
Mucositis	Altered oral mucous membranes Imbalanced nutrition: less than body requirements Acute pain
Multiorgan failure	Ineffective peripheral tissue/renal/gastrointestinal/cerebral perfusions Impaired gas exchange Activity intolerance Severe anxiety/fear Risk for infection Imbalanced nutrition: less than body requirements
Cardiac failure	Decreased cardiac output Excess fluid volume Risk for impaired gas exchange Activity intolerance Risk for impaired skin integrity

Data from Refs.[1,13,19–26]

- Diarrhea
- Jaundice

Specific Care

One of the most important HSCT care considerations is neutropenia and infection prevention. HSCT patients often have central lines that can be a source for infection. Many patients also experience mucositis and mouth sores from the chemotherapy regimens, which can be a portal for infections. The Centers for Disease Control and Prevention recently distinguished a difference between a central line infection and infection that originates from mucosal barrier injury.[31] Maintaining a high standard of practice in terms of infection prevention for this highly vulnerable population includes:

- Hand hygiene before and after entering a patient's room
- Central line dressing care
- Proper technique for central line blood draws

Diligence in these areas could reduce the risk of infection for HSCT patients.[31,32]

Communication

Communication with HSCT staff is especially important for non–HSCT-trained staff on general floors and staff in the ICU taking care of HSCT patients. Because these staff are usually unaccustomed to the unique patient care required, HSCT staff need to communicate the presence of many threats to this patient population. Care coordination and ongoing communication between the HSCT and ICU staff have been shown to improve continuity of care, clarification of goals, and establishment of resources for future questions,[5,13,33] which is especially important at each care transition. **Fig. 1** shows how HSCT nurses are the thread that connects multiple disciplines with HSCT patients and families. The gray arrow in the figure represents HSCT nurses using communication, education, support, and specific care of patients, families, and the nonspecialized staff through the care settings.

Support

Non–HSCT-trained staff and ICU staff need ongoing support by HSCT staff. Initial orientation for staff is essential; however, a need for ongoing education and practice updates in a variety of formats should be incorporated to stay current and maintain quality care.[18,33] Establishing resources at each care transition and being available to answer questions is a way to support staff caring for patients going through HSCT.

PATIENT INTERVENTIONS

Patient interventions following admission to the ICU revolve around communicating the prognosis, identifying which interventions are being implemented, incorporating

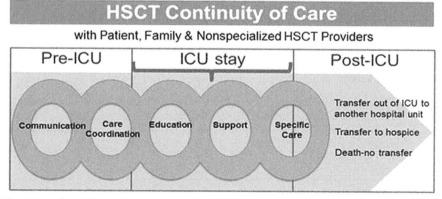

Fig. 1. Nursing influence on HSCT continuity of care.

patients in care planning, and educating patients on how they can assist in their care.[33]

Education and Specific Care

Education for patients who are in the ICU should revolve around prognosis and maintaining independence. Nursing staff should communicate the interventions the medical teams will do or have done and how they may affect care. Nursing staff should promote and educate patients on how to optimize independence with activities of daily living (ADLs). Encouraging independence, adequate nutrition, and physical exercise in the ICU can help support patients by being consistent with HSCT staff recommendations and prior education. Attention to how educational information is given should also be considered in terms of timing, patient readiness, and appropriate education level.[33] Including patients in care and educating them on ways to maintain self-care may be a valuable intervention in terms of patient safety, continuity, and quality of care.[33]

Communication

HSTC nursing staff can be the front-line communicators between ICU providers and patients. This role may include promoting patient involvement and provider transparency during rounds, encouraging patients to ask questions and voice their concerns about dying, or voice care preferences.[29] Staff can communicate to patients expected treatment progress and impact on outcomes. Communicating care preferences such as preferred supplemental nutrition is also a way for patients to maintain dignity and a sense of control. Communicating simple things to patients may seem minor; however, it has a large impact on the lived and perceived patient care experience.[29]

Support

Much like other ICU patients, HSCT patients are at risk for anxiety, death anxiety, and fear. Patients may or may not be physically or emotionally able to assist with appropriate tasks of self-care. However, giving them the opportunity to participate in care and care planning improves the quality of care and allows patients to express their feelings and feel useful.[33] Patients in the ICU are unfamiliar with care expectations and ICU routines. ICU staff can clarify expectations for patients to better know how and when to participate in care. Encouraging patients each day is a common intervention but one that should not be overlooked. Staff can work with patients to foster coping skills to rebalance thoughts around prior health status to present health.[34] Identifying available resources, including patients' own internal resources, such as innate personality and prior experiences with stress, and external resources, such as supportive family and friends, supports patients.[34] Working with patients to physically and emotionally adjust to their changed health statuses can help foster coping skills.

FAMILY INTERVENTIONS

For the purpose of this article, family members include caregivers and are referred to as family caregivers. Family is defined as people whom the patient identifies as family and not by a legal definition of family. Within the HSCT population, most caregivers are family.[29,30,35,36]

Specific Care

Family caregivers are essential to patient outcomes and the success of HSCT centers. Family caregivers are intricately involved in the patient's care and work as a liaison between the health care staff, the patient, and family at home. Because of the variety of HSCT infrastructure and differences in HSCT programs, caregiver responsibilities vary between each institution. Caregivers typically help with ADLs, medication management, meal preparation, and transportation. They also keep track of blood counts and provide status updates with distant family members and friends. Nurses who understand the unique role of the family caregiver for HSCT patients and facilitate them fulfilling their duties nurture the concept of continuity of care for each patient.

Education

Being a caregiver for someone going through HSCT is a dynamic process and demands both physical and emotional presence.[34] Many studies have investigated the physical, emotional, social, and spiritual effects of being a family caregiver and how it can affect sleep, anxiety, cognitive decline, and financial and caregiver burdens.[34,37] Preparation for the physical and psychological aspects of caregiving is essential because it allows caregivers the chance to learn and manage new information and practice new techniques. Without adequate education in preparation for their role, they are at increased risk of having negative effects from caregiving. Education inclusive of skill practice before assuming their role is a way to help prepare caregivers to be successful.

A transfer to the ICU may pose an abrupt break in family caregiver duties and caregivers may be at a loss for how to best help the patient in the new environment. Although some caregivers enjoy a reprieve in care, others may appreciate guidance and involvement with patient care activities of ADLs and mealtimes.

In addition, encouraging and offering opportunities for family caregivers to take care of their own health and maintain self-care is important not only for them but for the patients as well.[33] Caregivers often place the patient's needs ahead of their own, which puts them at risk for emotional and physical decline.[37] Educating caregivers on proper nutrition, sleep, and stress relief, as well as pointing out opportunities for breaks, are ways to support them while patients are in the ICU. Enforcing education previously given on the floor for skill mastery and self-care are also interventions for family members of patients going through HSCT.

Communication

ICU staff can involve family caregivers in patient care by communicating status updates, laboratory values, and next steps in care.[1] Family caregivers of HSCT patients are accustomed to working closely with HSCT teams and bringing this expectation of close and frequent communication with staff to the ICU setting. Family caregivers are also involved in communicating with other family members and friends. One study[29,30] found that encouragement to use websites such Caringbridge to keep the communication ongoing with others was effective. In addition, encouragement to ask for help, physician rounds with the patient and family caregivers present, open/honest communication inclusive of communication about dying, and asking questions are communication strategies that were found to be helpful.[29]

Support

In the ICU, staff can support family caregivers through validation, fostering coping and problem-solving skills, and encouraging self-care.[34,37] Recognizing that family caregivers are also managing finances, their homes, additional roles, changes, and uncertainty while the patient is in the ICU is key to their support as well.[29,30] Communicating to caregivers that they are doing a great job in providing support for their loved ones and acknowledging their contributions to patient care is an excellent a way to support them and show they are valued.

Staff can work with family caregivers to foster coping and problem-solving skills to rebalance thoughts around patients' prior health statuses and their present health states.[34] Staff can help identify available caregiver resources for family caregivers. Helping caregivers identify backup caregivers and incorporate family involvement so they can take a break is important.[37] Offering opportunities for family caregivers to take care of their own health, through mental or physical breaks, and maintain self-care is a way to support them. Preparing caregivers to effectively cope and problem solve can aid in communicating and interacting with the medical teams.

SUMMARY

The experience of being in the ICU environment, as a result of complications during and after the transplant or because of relapse, redefines the patient and family experience. With the anticipated growth of HSCT, understanding the adult HSCT patient and family caregiver experience in the ICU is necessary. There is a need for further research and practice improvement to address the unique care needs of HSCT patients and their caregivers. Identifying relevant medical and nursing diagnoses for this patient population is essential to that care. HSCT nurses play a role in supporting staff, patients, and caregivers while in the ICU through education about new expectations and prognoses, communication status updates, and support of coping and problem-solving skills. The importance of these interventions is unique to patients going through HSCT because of the intensity of treatment and the dynamic nature of the HSCT trajectory. Providing these interventions provides hope, clarifies goals, and unifies care in a time of uncertainty. Nurses specialized in HSCT care are key to connecting many disciplines with patients and their caregivers and coordinating care across multiple care settings. These nurses can help educate non–HSCT-trained staff, enhance communication with the ICU staff, and facilitate collaboration among the health care team members to ensure quality of care and improve outcomes for patients going through HSCT.

REFERENCES

1. Kasberg H, Brister L, Barnard B. Aggressive disease, aggressive treatment: the adult hematopoietic stem cell transplant patients in the intensive care unit. AACN Adv Crit Care 2011;22(4):349–64.
2. Pasquini MC, Zhu X. Current uses and outcomes of hematopoietic stem cell transplantation: CIBMTR summary slides. 2015. Available at: https://www.cibmtr.org.
3. Siegel RL, Miller KD, Jemal A. Cancer statistics, 2016. CA Cancer J Clin 2016;66: 7–30.
4. Health Resources and Services Administration. Blood cell transplant. 2016. Available at: http://bloodcell.transplant.hrsa.gov/index.html.
5. Jenkins P, Johnston LJ, Pickham D, et al. Intensive care utilization for hematopoietic cell transplant recipients. Biol Blood Marrow Transplant 2015;21(11):2023–7.
6. Lengline E, Chevret S, Moreau A-S, et al. Changes in intensive care for allogeneic hematopoietic stem cell transplant recipients. Bone Marrow Transplant 2015;50: 840–5.
7. Naeem N, Reed MD, Creger RJ, et al. Transfer of the hematopoietic stem cell transplant patient to the intensive care unit: does it really matter? Bone Marrow Transplant 2006;37(2):119–33.
8. Agarwal S, O'Donoghue S, Gowardman J, et al. Intensive care unit experience of haemopoietic stem cell transplant patients. Intern Med J 2012;42(7):748–54.

9. Bokhari SW, Munir T, Memon S, et al. Impact of critical care reconfiguration and track-and-trigger outreach team intervention on outcomes of haematology patients requiring intensive care admission. Ann Hematol 2010;89(5):505–12.

10. Geraghty K, Pascua R, Saria M. Improving the care of critically-ill hematopoietic stem cell transplant patients: challenges of a non-specialized nursing staff. Oncol Nurs Forum 2006;33(2):476.

11. Kew AK, Couban S, Patrick W, et al. Outcome of hematopoietic stem cell transplant recipients admitted to the intensive care unit. Biol Blood Marrow Transplant 2006;12(3):301–5.

12. Moreau AS, Seguin A, Lemiale V, et al. Survival and prognostic factors of allogeneic hematopoietic stem cell transplant recipients admitted to intensive care unit. Leuk Lymphoma 2014;55(6):1417–20.

13. Saria MG, Gosselin-Acomb TK. Hematopoietic stem cell transplantation: implications for critical care nurses. Clin J Oncol Nurs 2006;11(1):53–63.

14. Townsend WM, Holroyd A, Pearce R, et al. Improved intensive care unit survival for critically ill allogeneic haematopoietic stem cell transplant recipients following reduced intensity conditioning. Br J Haematol 2013;161(4):578–86.

15. Ezzone S, Schmit-Pokornyk K. Blood and marrow stem cell transplantation: principles, practice and nursing insights. 3rd edition. Sudbury (MA): Jones & Bartlett Publishers; 2007.

16. Glemser E, Lindsey S, Andres M. Meeting the needs of nurses new to oncology. Oncol Nurs Forum 2007;34(2):561.

17. Rees L, Sylvanus T. BMT core curriculum: evolution of education. Oncol Nurs Forum 2007;34(2):538–9.

18. Wickline M, Yanke R. Meeting the challenges of providing ongoing oncology nursing education: Puget Sound Oncology Nursing Education Cooperative. Oncol Nurs Forum 2007;34(2):297–9.

19. Herdman T, Kamitzuru S, editors. NANDA International, Inc. Nursing diagnoses: definitions & classification 2015-2017. 10th edition. Chichester, UK; Ames, IA: Wiley Blackwell; 2014.

20. Afessa B, Tefferi A, Dunn WF, et al. Intensive care unit support and Acute Physiology and Chronic Health Evaluation III performance in hematopoietic stem cell transplant recipients. Crit Care Med 2003;31(6):1715–21.

21. Doenges M, Moorhouse F, Murr A. In: Nursing diagnosis manual: planning, individualizing, and documenting client care. 5th edition. Philadelphia: FA Davis Company; 2016.

22. Gilbert C, Vasu T, Baram M. Use of mechanical ventilation and renal replacement therapy in critically ill hematopoietic stem cell transplant recipients. Biol Blood Marrow Transplant 2013;19(2):321–4.

23. McArdle J. Critical care outcomes in the hematologic transplant recipient. Clin Chest Med 2009;30(1):155–67.

24. Saillard C, Blaise D, Mokart D. Critically ill allogeneic hematopoietic stem cell transplantation patients in the intensive care unit: reappraisal of actual prognosis. Bone Marrow Transplant 2016;51:1050–61.

25. Scales D, Thiruchelvan D, Kiss A, et al. Intensive care outcomes in bone marrow transplant recipients: a population-based cohort analysis. Crit Care 2008;12(3):R77.

26. Sosa E. Veno-occlusive disease in hematopoietic stem cell transplantations recipients. Clin J Oncol Nurs 2012;16(5):507–13.

27. Cooke L, Gemmill R, Grant L. Creating a palliative educational session for hematopoietic stem cell transplantation recipients at relapse. Clin J Oncol Nurs 2011;15(4):411–7.

28. Young L, Polzin J, Todd S, et al. Validation of the nursing diagnosis anxiety in adult patients undergoing bone marrow transplant. Int J Nurs Terminol Classif 2002;13(3):88–100.

29. Young L. The family experience following bone marrow/blood cell transplantation. Dissertation 2010;19(2):1–196.

30. Young L. The family experience following bone marrow/blood cell transplantation. J Adv Nurs 2013;69(10):2274–84.

31. Ruefer KE, Murray T, Black L, et al. Nursing education regarding identification, assessment, and treatment of mucositis in inpatient oncology. Biol Blood Marrow Transplant 2016;22(3):S467–8.

32. Bevans M, Tierney DK, Bruch C, et al. Hematopoietic stem cell transplantation nursing: a practice variation study. Oncol Nurs Forum 2009;36(6):E317–25.

33. Thomson B, Gorospe G, Cooke L, et al. Transitions of care: a hematopoietic stem cell transplantation nursing education project across the trajectory. Clin J Oncol Nurs 2015;19(4):E74–9.

34. Gemmill R, Cooke L, Williams AC, et al. Informal caregivers of hematopoietic cell transplant patients: a review and recommendations for interventions and research. Cancer Nurs 2011;34(6):E13–21.

35. Williams L. Informal caregiving dynamics with a case study in blood and marrow transplantation. Oncol Nurs Forum 2003;30(4):679–89.

36. Frey P, Stinson T, Siston A, et al. Lack of caregivers limits use of outpatient hematopoietic stem cell transplant program. Bone Marrow Transplant 2002; 30(11):741–8.

37. Beattie S, Lebel S. The experience of caregivers of hematological cancer patients undergoing a hematopoietic stem cell transplant: a comprehensive literature review. Psychooncology 2011;20:1137–50.

Coagulopathy In and Outside the Intensive Care Unit

 CrossMark

Marie Bashaw, DNP, RN, NEA-BC

KEYWORDS

- Coagulopathy • ICU • Sepsis • Acute traumatic coagulopathy

KEY POINTS

- Coagulopathy is life threatening.
- Through technological advances of today, early recognition of the signs and symptoms of coagulopathy and the complicating factors is possible in most settings.
- By implementing appropriate treatment modalities early, the progression of coagulopathy can be halted, reducing morbidity and mortality.

INTRODUCTION

Coagulopathy occurs both inside and outside the intensive care unit (ICU). Early recognition of this condition is essential in the care and treatment of these patients. Coagulopathy is a disease or condition affecting the blood's ability to coagulate.[1] This bleeding disorder is a major contributor to morbidity and mortality. Many factors contribute to coagulopathy, including acidosis, blood loss, hypothermia, hemodilution, consumption and dilution of coagulation factors, tissue trauma, and shock.[2,3] When there is prolongation of prothrombin time (PT) greater than 18 s and activated partial thromboplastin time (APTT) greater than 60 s, coagulopathy occurs.[2] Without treatment, coagulopathy is life threatening (**Fig. 1**).

Coagulopathy is precipitated via several different mechanisms. This article presents the continuum of coagulopathy and interventions necessary to treat this deadly event in illness.

COAGULOPATHY OF CRITICAL ILLNESS
Sepsis

In septic patients, a key event leading to coagulopathy is the body's overwhelming response to a pathogen, leading to an overexpression of the inflammatory system.[4]

College of Nursing and Health, Wright State University, 3640 Colonel Glenn Highway, Dayton, OH 45435, USA
E-mail address: Marie.bashaw@wright.edu

Crit Care Nurs Clin N Am 29 (2017) 353–362
http://dx.doi.org/10.1016/j.cnc.2017.04.005
0899-5885/17/© 2017 Elsevier Inc. All rights reserved.

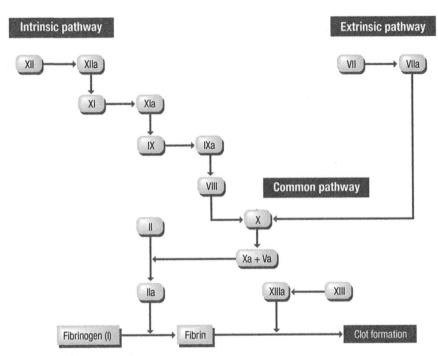

Fig. 1. Coagulation cascade.

Hypercoagulation occurs initially, leading to the formation of microthrombi. Microthrombi cause vascular occlusion and cell death, which result in multiorgan failure. In the late stages of sepsis, hypocoagulation results in the uncontrolled consumption of platelets and coagulation factors.[5] Microvascular breakdown leads to organ failure and death, disseminated intravascular coagulation (DIC).[5] Treatment of the underlying pathogen is essential. In addition to sepsis, another cause of coagulopathy is major trauma.

Trauma

Acute traumatic coagulopathy (ATC) is the leading cause of death in trauma victims as a result of uncontrolled bleeding and exsanguination. Risk factors for trauma-induced coagulopathy include metabolic acidosis, hypothermia, hypoperfusion, hemodilution, and fluid replacement.[6,7] In a consumptive coagulopathy, fibrinogen and factor V are the most depleted clotting factors.[8]

When tissue trauma and inflammation occur, hypothermia and shock ensue. Hypothermia worsens coagulopathy by inducing hepatic sequestration of platelets, reducing platelet function, and decreasing rate of fibrin formation,[9] resulting in a weak, slowly formed clot that is inadequate for hemostasis.[10] Fewer than 9% of trauma patients are hypothermic on presentation, so aggressive measures to prevent radiant heat loss during resuscitation are indicated.[11]

Hypothermia, acidosis, and hemodilution lead to activation of the endothelium and the release of heparin-like substances that impair the body's ability to clot.[7] This potentiates the coagulopathy spiral that is complicated by hemodilution from aggressive volume resuscitation. Left untreated, ATC results in death.

Obstetric Disseminated Intravascular Coagulation

Coagulopathy differs from the presentation of coagulopathy in emergency department or ICU patients. Coagulopathy in obstetric patients is caused massive obstructive trauma. Massive obstetric trauma caused by placenta abruption, placenta previa, placenta accreta, and postpartum hemorrhage is the leading cause of maternal morbidity and mortality.[12,13] The 4 Ts – tone, tissues, trauma, and thrombin – are potential causes of postpartum hemorrhage. Early recognition and prompt treatment are necessary in managing massive obstetric hemorrhage. During placental abruption, massive amounts of fibrinogen are lost resulting in thrombocytopenia.[12] Volume replacement for postpartum hemorrhage can also cause coagulopathy secondary to the dilution of coagulation factors. Proper treatment is essential in the prevention of maternal morbidity and mortality. Another cause of coagulopathy is hepatic insufficiency.

Hepatic Insufficiency

Chronic liver insufficiency and failure lead to portal hypertension, hypersplenism, thrombocytopenia, and gastroesophageal varices, each of which is associated with increased bleeding risk.[14] Hemostasis is impacted by liver disease. The liver plays a prominent role in the synthesis of coagulation factors and reduction of procoagulant and anticoagulant factors, fibrinolytic factors, and antifibrinolytic proteins.[14] Because all procoagulant factors except factor VIII occur in the liver, when hepatic insufficiency is present, hemorrhage and coagulopathy are significant risks.

Cardiopulmonary Bypass

Coagulopathy contributes to significant blood loss in some cardiac surgery patients,[15,16] resulting in the need for administration of blood products in as many as 50% of patients.[17,18] There are 3 major factors that contribute to bleeding in the cardiac surgery patient. First, the extracorporeal circuit used during cardiopulmonary bypass requires high doses of heparin to keep the bypass circuit from clotting. Second, shed blood in the surgical field becomes a major source of thrombin generation.[19] Washing of blood shed from the surgical field removes all platelets and clotting factors as well as tissue factor, which can result in further clotting activation.[20] Third, platelets are partially activated during cardiopulmonary bypass, either by thrombin or some other mechanism that prevents them from fully activating when needed to control hemostasis postoperatively.[21]

MEDICATION-INDUCED COAGULOPATHY

Although anticoagulant medications provide protection from thrombotic events, these agents are also associated with increased risk for severe bleeding with injury. For example, anticoagulant therapy in the presence of intracranial hemorrhage, whether spontaneous or traumatic, may become a life-threatening coagulopathy.[22] Guidelines on holding anticoagulant medications for planned procedures as well as protocols for urgent reversal are discussed later.

CONGENITAL COAGULOPATHY

Hemangiomas, hemophilia A and hemophilia B, and von Willebrand disease type 3 are congenital coagulopathy conditions. The most common hepatic tumor in infants is a hepatic hemangioma. Although most hepatic hemangiomas in infants undergo spontaneous resorption, some hepatic hemangiomas can be life threatening when hemorrhage or consumptive coagulopathy occurs from tumor rupture.[23] Hemophilia, a rare genetic disease linked to the X chromosome, results in the inability to produce clotting factors needed to stop bleeding. Hemophilia A is a deficiency in clotting factor VIII and hemophilia B is a deficiency in clotting factor IX.[24] von Willebrand disease, the most common inherited bleeding disorder, is an autosomal inherited disorder affecting women and men equally. Women are impacted more through hemostatic challenges with menstrual bleeding and childbirth.[25]

DIAGNOSIS/TECHNIQUES
Plasma-Based Coagulation Assays

Coagulopathy is a complex process to diagnose. At this point, there is no universally accepted blood test to define the extent of a coagulopathy, but most clinicians agree that an elevated prothrombin time (PT)/international normalized ratio (INR) indicates that a coagulopathy is present.[8] Standard coagulation tests, such as PT/INR, aPTT, and fibrinogen level, were originally designed to monitor congenital single-factor clotting deficiencies rather than multiple factor–acquired coagulopathies and are not reliable predictors of bleeding in these patients because the test does not account platelet function, fibrinolytic activity, or thrombin generation.[26] Plasma-based coagulation assays, however, do have an important role in guiding use of blood products in the management of ongoing bleeding.[8]

Viscoelastic Hemostatic Assays

For trauma patients with moderate to severe coagulopathies, viscoelastic hemostatic assays provide guidance in resuscitation with blood products.[27,28] They are particularly useful in situations when both the clot formation and clot degradation are occurring simultaneously, such as in DIC. Hyperfibrinolysis occurs when the rate of fibrin degradation exceeds the rate of fibrin formation, resulting in compromised clot strength.[29]

These tests are less useful in minimally injured patients, because patients tend to have normal coagulation profiles.[27,30] Another limitation of thromboelastography (TEG; TEM Systems, Inc, Durham, NC) and rotational thromboelastometry (ROTEM; TEM International GmbH, Munich, Germany) is that they do not detect the impact of antiplatelet therapy.[31]

PROGNOSIS/CLINICAL MANAGEMENT: BLOOD PRODUCTS

In the management of traumatic coagulopathy, the United States tends to use fresh frozen plasma (FFP), whereas European countries tend to use fibrinogen concentrates in combination with other synthetic clotting factor products.[8] Fibrogen concentrate (Haemocomplettan, CSL Behring, Marburg, Germany) was originally approved for congenital fibrinogen deficiency but is used off-label to treat massive bleeding.[32,33]

In cardiac surgery patients, the primary blood products used to manage postoperative bleeding are FFP, cryoprecipitate, and platelets, but large volumes are needed to achieve an acceptable replacement of depleted clotting factors.[34] Cryoprecipitate is given to increase fibrinogen levels; however, there is not a clear fibrinogen level to trigger administration because baseline fibrinogen levels vary widely.[35]

Platelet replacement is indicated when the total platelet count is less than $185 \times 10^3/\mu L$[36] and in the presence of antiplatelet therapy.[37] In traumatic coagulopathy, platelets become unresponsive to activating factors,[38] which may explain improved patient outcomes when platelet transfusion occurs in the presence of adequate platelet counts.[39,40] In addition, the quality of transfused platelets matters because patients may be deficient in endogenous platelet activating factors.[41]

REVERSAL AGENTS
Antiplatelet Drugs

Aspirin and clopidogrel (Plavix, Bristol-Myers Squibb and Sanofi Pharmaceuticals partnership, Bridgewater, New Jersey) are antiplatelet drugs. Several newer antiplatelet drugs include prasugrel (Effient, Eli Lilly and Company, Indianapolis, Indiana), ticagrelor (Brilinta, AstraZeneca, Boston, MA), and cilostazol (Pletal, Cadila Pharmaceuticals, Ahmedabad, Gujarat), used with high-risk patients in percutaneous coronary procedures to prevent stenosis or occlusion.[42]

$P2Y_{12}$ inhibitors, such as clopidogrel, increase the risk of postoperative bleeding and the need for blood product administration.[43] The current recommendation by the Society of Thoracic Surgeons (2012) is to delay surgery for 5 days to 7 days to hold $P2Y_{12}$ inhibitors. Aspirin can be continued as a bridge to prevent thrombotic cardiac events while waiting for surgery. Platelet transfusion is indicated for urgent reversal, because there are no reversal agents for antiplatelet drugs.[37] In severe cases of intracranial bleeding related to antiplatelet drugs, desmopressin acetate may be given in addition to the platelet transfusion to increase platelet activation.[22]

Heparin and Heparinoids

Heparin and heparinoids increase the activity of antithrombin III, which inactivates thrombin, plasmin, and the activated forms of factors IX, X, XI, and XII. The recommended reversal agent for heparin and low-molecular-weight heparin is protamine, although protamine is less successful at reversing low-molecular-weight heparin so severe cases may require administration of factor VIIa.[44] The recommended laboratory tests to assess effectiveness of therapy and reversal agents are aPTT or anti–factor Xa.[44]

Warfarin

Warfarin antagonizes vitamin K–dependent production of clotting factors II, VII, IX, and X. Dietary consumption of vitamin K counteracts warfarin, which drives the variance in effects of warfarin therapy, which requires regular blood monitoring. The recommended laboratory test to assess effectiveness of both therapy and reversal agent is the PT, which is more commonly expressed as INR. Holding warfarin for 3 days to 5 days, either with or without concurrent administration of vitamin K, prior to an invasive procedure is recommended.[45] For urgent reversal of warfarin, the administration of prothrombin complex concentrate (PCC) is recommended.[44]

Novel Oral Anticoagulants

Novel oral anticoagulants (NOACs), which offer an alternative to warfarin therapy, can result in excessive bleeding in acute trauma patients or in surgical patients who have not received sufficient advice, or complied with the advice, on stopping these medications before major surgery.[31] There are 2 types of NOAC: direct factor Xa inhibitors (eg, apixaban and rivaroxaban) and direct thrombin inhibitors (eg, dabigatran). There is no therapeutic laboratory monitoring test established for either direct factor Xa inhibitors or direct thrombin inhibitors.

Because there are few research data on the reversal of NOACs in bleeding patients after cardiopulmonary bypass,[46] the current recommendation is to stop NOACs at least 3 days before cardiac surgery.[31] There are no specific reversal agents for NOACs, which leaves the most effective reversal strategy the administration of

PCC.[47,48] There are promising studies on the effectiveness of factor eight inhibitor bypassing activity in reversal the action of direct thrombin inhibitors.[49] There is a reversal agent for dabigatran, idarucizumab (Praxbind, Boehringer Ingelheim, Germany). This is a monoclonal antibody fragment that reduces the level of unbound dabigatran in the blood stream and normalizes coagulation parameters.[50]

CONTROVERSIES
Point-of-Care Testing

One concern about the usefulness of point-of-care testing for clotting times is the time involved. Plasma-based coagulation assays, such as PT/INR, require significant turn-around time, which can delay the immediate management of an ATC.[8] Viscoelastic hemostatic assays, such as ROTEM and TEG, may be predictive of transfusion requirements, but there is a lack of randomized trials to validate this use.[8] Viscoelastic assays also require significant turnaround time, although preliminary decisions can be made based on the data from the early phase of clot formation.

There is no single laboratory test that can consistently guide management of bleeding. For example, a consumptive coagulopathy that occurs in traumatic injury is indicated by elevated clotting times (PT/INR and aPTT), high thrombin-generating capacity, and reduced platelet counts.[8] But in cardiac surgery patients, fibrinogen level may be the best coagulation factor to predict of the severity of postoperative bleeding.[51] Rather than looking for a single indicator, it is more helpful to evaluate multiple indictors to determine the cause and extent of the coagulopathy.

Tranexamic Acid

Tranexamic acid (TXA) inhibits activation of plasminogen to plasmin, which is a fibrinolytic protein. The CRASH-2 trial of trauma patients resulted in one-third reduction in mortality due to hemorrhage when patients received TXA.[52] TXA has also been shown to reduce postoperative bleeding in cardiac surgery patients due to hyperfibrinolysis, which occurs in approximately 6% to 8% of patients experiencing postoperative bleeding.[53]

Single-Factor Therapy

Originally developed for hemophilia, recombinant factor VIIa (NovoSeven, Novo Nordisk, Bagsvaerd, Denmark) has been used off-label for treatment of ATC for some time in Europe.[54] The early research on the risk of using recombinant factor VIIa in trauma patients is that there is no difference in thromboembolic events compared with placebo.[55]

Massive Transfusion Protocols

The recent military experience in Iraq and Afghanistan has provided greater understanding of the role of ATC in traumatic death, leading to improved outcomes in patients treated hemostatic resuscitation either with fresh whole blood[56] or a balanced mix of red blood cells, FFP, and platelets (sometimes with the addition of cryoprecipitate or TXA) coupled with the extremely limited use of crystalloid infusions.[57–59]

The current Trauma Quality Improvement Program guidelines from the American College of Surgeons (2016) distinguishes between massive transfusion in the resuscitation bay (emergency room, operating room, or angiography suite) from massive transfusion in the ICU. During the resuscitation phase, crystalloid solutions are avoided in favor of universal blood products that are transfused in a 1:1:1 ratio (equal parts) of red blood cells, plasma, and platelets. Once bleeding has been controlled, the patient moves into the critical care phase with a laboratory-based transfusion algorithm based on PT/INR, aPTT, fibrinogen level, hemoglobin/hematocrit, platelet count, and viscoelastic hemostatic assays, if available. It is important to note that it is the cessation of uncontrolled bleeding that marks the transition from the resuscitative phase to the critical care phase and not a patient's physical location.

Balanced transfusion strategies, such as 1:1:1, still result in hemodilution due to the presence of anticoagulants and additives in the stored blood products, resulting in decreased effectiveness of both platelets and clotting factors.[8] Massive transfusion may lead to volume overload, increasing the risk of mortality from adult respiratory distress syndrome and multisystem organ failure.[58]

SUMMARY

Coagulopathy is life threatening. Through technological advances of today, early recognition of the signs and symptoms of coagulopathy and the complicating factors is possible in most settings. By implementing appropriate treatment modalities early, the progression coagulopathy can be halted, which reduces morbidity and mortality.

REFERENCES

1. Coagulopathy. Merriam-Webster; 2016. Available at: https://www.merriam-webster.com.
2. Kaczynski J, Wilczynska M, Fligelstone L, et al. The pathophysiology, diagnosis and treatment of the acute coagulopathy of trauma and shock: a literature review. Eur J Trauma Emerg Surg 2015;41(3):259–72.
3. Sorensen B, Fries D. Emerging treatment strategies for trauma-induced coagulopathy. Br J Surg 2012;99:40–50.
4. Semeraro N, Ammollo C, Semeraro F, et al. Coagulopathy of acute sepsis. Semin Thromb Hemost 2015;41(6):650–8.
5. Johansen M, Jensen J, Johansson P, et al. Regular article: mild induced hypothermia: effects on sepsis-related coagulopathy -results from a randomized controlled trial. Thromb Res 2015;135:175–82.
6. Katrancha E, Gonzalez Iii L. Trauma-induced coagulopathy. Crit Care Nurse 2014;34(4):54–63.
7. Maegele M. The coagulopathy of trauma. Eur J Trauma Emerg Surg 2014;40(2):113–26.
8. Cap A, Hunt B. The pathogenesis of traumatic coagulopathy. Anaesthesia 2015;70(Suppl 1):96–101.
9. Watts D, Trask A, Soeken K, et al. Hypothermic coagulopathy in trauma: effect of varying levels of hypothermia on enzyme speed, platelet function, and fibrinolytic activity. J Trauma 1998;44(5):846–54.
10. Dirkmann D, Hanke A, Görlinger K, et al. Hypothermia and acidosis synergistically impair coagulation in human whole blood. Anesth Analg 2008;106(6):1627–32.
11. Tsuei B, Kearney P. Hypothermia in the trauma patient. Injury 2004;35(1):7.
12. Collis R, Collins P. Haemostatic management of obstetric haemorrhage. Anaesthesia 2015;70(Suppl 1):78–86.
13. Su LL, Chong YS. Massive obstetric haemorrhage with disseminated intravascular coagulopathy. Best Pract Res Clin Obstet Gynaecol 2012;26(1):77–90.
14. Barton C. Treatment of coagulopathy related to hepatic insufficiency. Crit Care Med 2016;44(10):1927–33.

15. Andreasen J, Nielsen C. Prophylactic tranexamic acid in elective, primary coronary artery bypass surgery using cardiopulmonary bypass. Eur J Cardiothorac Surg 2004;26(2):311–7.

16. Chu M, Wilson S, Novick R, et al. Original article: cardiovascular: does clopidogrel increase blood loss following coronary artery bypass surgery? Ann Thorac Surg 2004;78:1536–41.

17. Bennett-Guerrero E, Song H, O'Brien S, et al. Temporal changes in the use of blood products for coronary artery bypass graft surgery in North America: an analysis of the Society of Thoracic surgeons adult cardiac database. J Cardiothorac Vasc Anesth 2010;24(5):814–6.

18. Ferraris V, Brown J, Shann K, et al. Special report: STS workforce on evidence based surgery: 2011 update to the Society of Thoracic Surgeons and the Society of cardiovascular anesthesiologists blood conservation clinical practice guidelines* *The International Consortium for evidence based perfusion formally endorses these guidelines. Ann Thorac Surg 2011;91:944–82.

19. Chung J, Gikakis N, Rao A, et al. Pericardial blood activates the extrinsic coagulation pathway during clinical cardiopulmonary bypass. Circulation 1996;93(11):2014–8.

20. De Somer F, Van Belleghem Y, Van Nooten G, et al. Cardiopulmonary support and physiology (CSP): tissue factor as the main activator of the coagulation system during cardiopulmonary bypass. J Thorac Cardiovasc Surg 2002;123:951–8.

21. Bevan D. Cardiac bypass haemostasis: putting blood through the mill. Br J Haematol 1999;104(2):208–19.

22. Medow JE, Dierks MR, Williams E, et al. The emergent reversal of coagulopathies encountered in neurosurgery and neurology: a technical note. Clin Med Res 2015;13(1):20–31.

23. Aslan H, Dural O, Yildirim G, et al. Prenatal diagnosis of a liver cavernous hemangioma. Fetal Pediatr Pathol 2013;32(5):341–5.

24. Rocha P, Carvalho M, Lopes M, et al. Costs and utilization of treatment in patients with hemophilia. BMC Health Serv Res 2015;15:484.

25. Govorov I, Ekrlund L, Mints M, et al. Heavy menstrual bleeding and health-associated quality of life in women with von Willebrand's disease. Exp Ther Med 2016;11(5):1923–9.

26. Dzik WH. Predicting hemorrhage using preoperative coagulation screening assays. Curr Hematol Rep 2004;3:324–30.

27. Kashuk J, Moore E, Sauaia A, et al. Primary fibrinolysis is integral in the pathogenesis of the acute coagulopathy of trauma. Ann Surg 2010;252(3):434–44.

28. Schochl H, Nienaber U, Solomon C, et al. Goal-directed coagulation management of major trauma patients using thromboelastometry (ROTEM (R))-guided administration of fibrinogen concentrate and prothrombin complex concentrate. Crit Care 2010;14(2). p. R55.

29. Hunt B, Segal H. Hyperfibrinolysis. J Clin Pathol 1996;49(12):958.

30. Rugeri L, Levrat A, Negrier C, et al. Diagnosis of early coagulation abnormalities in trauma patients by rotation thrombelastography. J Thromb Haemost 2007;5(2):289–95.

31. Davidson S. State of the Art - How I manage coagulopathy in cardiac surgery patients. Br J Haematol 2014;164(6):779–89.

32. Karlsson M, Ternström L, Jeppsson A, et al. Prophylactic fibrinogen infusion reduces bleeding after coronary artery bypass surgery. A prospective randomised pilot study. Thromb Haemost 2009;102(1):137–44.

33. Rahe-Meyer N, Pichlmaier M, Tanaka K, et al. Bleeding management with fibrinogen concentrate targeting a high-normal plasma fibrinogen level: a pilot study. Br J Anaesth 2009;102(6):785–92.
34. Chowdary P, Saayman A, Paulus U, et al. Efficacy of standard dose and 30 ml/kg fresh frozen plasma in correcting laboratory parameters of haemostasis in critically ill patients. Br J Haematol 2004;125(1):69–73.
35. Sørensen B, Bevan D. A critical evaluation of cryoprecipitate for replacement of fibrinogen. Br J Haematol 2010;149(6):834–43.
36. Hendrickson J, Shaz B, Josephson C, et al. Original article: coagulopathy is prevalent and associated with adverse outcomes in transfused pediatric trauma patients. J Pediatr 2012;160:204–9.e3.
37. Beshay J, Morgan H, Madden C, et al. Emergency reversal of anticoagulation and antiplatelet therapies in neurosurgical patients A review. J Neurosurg 2010;112(2):307–18.
38. Kutcher M, Redick B, Cohen M, et al. Characterization of platelet dysfunction after trauma. J Trauma Acute Care Surg 2012;73(1):13–9.
39. Perkins J, Cap A, Holcomb J, et al. Comparison of platelet transfusion as fresh whole blood versus apheresis platelets for massively transfused combat trauma patients (CME). Transfusion 2011;51(2):242–52.
40. Zink K, Sambasivan C, Holcomb J, et al. The North Pacific Surgical association: a high ratio of plasma and platelets to packed red blood cells in the first 6 hours of massive transfusion improves outcomes in a large multicenter study. Am J Surg 2009;197(Papers from the North Pacific Surgical Association):565–70.
41. Inaba K, Branco B, Demetriades D, et al. Impact of the duration of platelet storage in critically ill trauma patients. J Trauma 2011;71(6):1766–73.
42. Ju-Youn K, Yun-Seok C, Seung K, et al. It is not mandatory to use triple rather than dual anti-platelet therapy after a percutaneous coronary intervention with a second-generation drug-eluting stent. Medicine 2015;94(46):1–5.
43. Dunning J, Versteegh M, Nashef S, et al. Guideline on antiplatelet and anticoagulation management in cardiac surgery. Eur J Cardiothoracic Surg 2008;34(1): 73–92.
44. Imberti D, Barillari G, Ageno W, et al. Emergency reversal of anticoagulation with a three-factor prothrombin complex concentrate in patients with intracranial haemorrhage. Blood Transfus 2011;9(2):148–55.
45. Garcia D. Parenteral anticoagulants: antithrombotic therapy and prevention of thrombosis, 9th ed: American college of chest physicians evidence-based clinical practice guidelines (vol. 141, pg e24S, 2012). Chest 2012;144(2):721.
46. Warkentin T, Margetts P, Connolly S, et al. Recombinant factor Vila (rFVIIa) and hemodialysis to manage massive dabigatran-associated postcardiac surgery bleeding. Blood 2012;119(9):2172–4.
47. Eerenberg ES, Kamphuisen PW, Sijpkens MK, et al. Reversal of rivaroxaban and dabigatran by prothrombin complex concentrate: a randomized, placebo-controlled, crossover study in healthy subjects. Circulation 2011;124:1573–9.
48. Weitz JI, Quinlan DJ, Eikelboom JW. Periprocedural management and approach to bleeding in patients taking dabigatran. Circulation 2012;126:2428–32.
49. Khoo TL, Weatherburn C, Kershaw G, et al. The use of FEIBA® in the correction of coagulation abnormalities induced by induced by dabigatran. Int J Lab Hematol 2013;35:222–4.
50. Aschenbrenner D. Praxbind available as antidote to bleeding from pradaxa. Am J Nurs 2016;116(6):22–3.

51. Kozek-Langenecker S, Sorensen B, Hess J, et al. Clinical effectiveness of fresh frozen plasma compared with fibrinogen concentrate: a systematic review. Crit Care 2011;15(5):R239.

52. CRASH-2 collaborators, Roberts I, Shakur H, et al. The importance of early treatment with tranexamic acid in bleeding trauma patients: an exploratory analysis of the CRASH-2 randomised controlled trial. Lancet 2011;377(9771):1096–101.

53. Brenner B. Fibrinolysis in cardiac surgery management of bleeding after cardiac surgery. In: Mohr R, Goor DA, Lavee J, editors. Landes biosciences. Austin (TX): Landes Bioscience; 1997. p. 23–33.

54. Stein D, Dutton R, Alexander C, et al. Original scientific article: use of recombinant factor VIIa to facilitate organ donation in trauma patients with devastating neurologic injury. J Am Coll Surg 2009;208:120–5.

55. Boffard K, Riou B, Kluger Y, et al. Recombinant factor VIIa as adjunctive therapy for bleeding control in severely injured trauma patients: two parallel randomized, placebo-controlled, double-blind clinical trials. J Trauma 2005;59(1):8–18.

56. Spinella P, Holcomb J. Resuscitation and transfusion principles for traumatic hemorrhagic shock. Blood Rev 2009;23(6):231–40.

57. Borgman M, Spinella P, Holcomb J, et al. The ratio of blood products transfused affects mortality in patients receiving massive transfusions at a combat support hospital. J Trauma 2007;63(4):805–13.

58. Spahn D, Bouillon B, Rossaint R, et al. Management of bleeding and coagulopathy following major trauma: an updated European guideline. Crit Care 2013; 17(2):R76.

59. Callum J, Rizoli S. Assessment and management of massive bleeding: coagulation assessment, pharmacologic strategies, and transfusion management. Hematol Am Soc Hematol Educ Program 2012;2012:522–8.

Hidden Anemias in the Critically Ill

Patricia O'Malley, PhD, RN, APRN-CNS[a,b,*]

KEYWORDS

- Bloodless medicine • Erythropoietin-stimulating agents • Heart failure • Anemia

KEY POINTS

- With increasing knowledge of the risks associated with receiving blood transfusions, a new paradigm of bloodless medicine is needed.
- Principals of bloodless medicine include careful monitoring for obvious and hidden anemias, rapid intervention, minimizing blood losses from laboratory testing and procedures, and careful management of bleeding diatheses.
- As evidence is revealed and refined, standard treatment of anemia in the intensive care unit will include erythropoietin-stimulating agents, iron, folate, and vitamin B12, which will reduce risks associated with blood transfusions.

Nearly 70% of patients in the intensive care unit (ICU) for 1 week or longer will have a transfusion despite risks for infection and immune reactions.[1] Every unit unfused is correlated with a longer length of stay and increased risk of mortality.[2] Anemia is a symptom related to obvious and hidden causes described in **Table 1**.[1]

Anemia in heart failure (HF) and coronary heart disease reduces cardiac function and quality of life and increases hospital readmission rates.[3] Anemia is also associated with cognitive decline, weakening mobility, kidney injury and kidney disease progression, and poor graft outcomes in transplant.[4,5]

What does the evidence suggest? First, anemia in critical illness does not receive appropriate clinical attention, detection, management, and evaluation.[4] Even for the HF population, approximately 12% to 55% of patients have significant anemia from obvious and hidden causes.[5] Particularly at risk are elderly with unexplained anemia related to a limited response to endogenous erythropoietin.[4] Also unknown is whether anemia is responsible for poorer outcomes in HF or a symptom of disease progression. What is known is that anemia is linked with poorer outcomes and has multiple options for treatment.[3]

[a] Department of Nursing Research, Premier Health, Center of Nursing Excellence, 1 Wyoming Street, Dayton, OH 45409, USA; [b] School of Nursing, Indiana University East, 2325 Chester Boulevard, Richmond, IN 47374, USA
* Department of Nursing Research, Premier Health, Center of Nursing Excellence, 1 Wyoming Street, Dayton, OH 45409.
E-mail address: pomalley@premierhealth.com

Crit Care Nurs Clin N Am 29 (2017) 363–368
http://dx.doi.org/10.1016/j.cnc.2017.04.008
0899-5885/17/© 2017 Elsevier Inc. All rights reserved.

Table 1
Obvious and hidden sources of anemia in critically ill

Obvious	Hidden
• Gastrointestinal bleeding	• ↓ Erythropoietic response
• Coagulopathy	• ↑ Inflammatory cytokines
• Blood sampling	• ↓ Tumor necrosis factor
• Volume overload	• Iron malabsorption
• Aspirin	• Heme synthesis impairment
• Anticoagulants	• Iron deficiency
• Chronic kidney disease	• Nutritional deficits
• Procedural	• Medication side effects
• Laboratory testing	• Folate deficiency

Data from Jelkmann I, Jelkmann W. Impact of erythropoietin on intensive care patients. Transfus Med Hemother 2013;40:310–8; and Shander A, Goodnough LT, Javidroozi M, et al. Iron deficiency anemia-bridging the knowledge and practice gap. Transfus Med Rev 2014;28(3):156–66.

Treatment begins with assessment based on hemoglobin concentration and hematocrit level.[1] Other tools can include mean corpuscular volume, followed by biochemical analysis including transferrin saturation (iron adequacy to make red blood cells), and serum ferritin (stored iron). Iron deficiency (absolute or functional) is usually found with anemia.[4]

Medication history should never be overlooked in assessing anemia. **Table 2** describes common types of drug-induced anemia.[4,6–10]

Megaloblastic anemia, a type of macrocytic anemia usually related to vitamin B12 or vitamin B9 (folate) deficiency, may have origins in drug therapy as well. Certain drugs can interfere with absorption, transport, and delivery of vitamins or interrupt crucial biochemical processes and even destroy the vitamins. Implicated medications come from a variety of drug classes including antimalarial, antineoplastic, antibiotics, anticonvulsants, H2 blockers, and proton pump inhibitors. Other culprits can include allopurinol, alcohol, birth control, metformin, and gadolinium, a contrast agent used in MRI. For patients with this type of anemia, medication assessment is crucial to determine if drug therapy is the basis of the anemia.[11]

TREATMENT WITHOUT TRANSFUSION

The prevalence of anemia in the critically ill patient is significant, and the most common treatment is blood transfusion. Another option is erythropoietin-stimulating agents (ESAs) used off label. Commonly prescribed for patients with anemia related to end-stage renal disease, human immunodeficiency virus infection, and chemotherapy in nonmyeloid cancers, ESAs are also occasionally used preoperatively for major surgery (excluding heart surgery) to reduce transfusion burden.[12] Other off-label use includes treatment of anemia-related rheumatoid arthritis, lupus, or inflammatory bowel disease and in patients with reduced available iron. Use of ESAs in the ICU has been usually confined to patients with renal disease and approved indications and for Jehovah Witnesses who refuse allogeneic blood transfusions.[1]

Drugs in the ESA class are epoetin alfa (marketed as Epogen [Amgen, Thousand Oaks, CA] and Procrit [Janssen, Titusville, NJ]) and darbepoetin alfa (marketed as Aranesp [Amgen, Thousand Oaks, CA]) and stimulate the bone marrow to produce red blood cells. Response to ESAs is often diminished because of the inflammatory responses of critical illness. As a result, higher doses of ESAs (compared with doses for chronic kidney disease patients) are required to overcome the inhibition exerted

Table 2
Potential drug-induced anemias: type and possible medications

Anemia Type	Medications
Hemolytic *Premature destruction of erythrocytes and bone marrow activity unable to compensate for erythrocyte loss. Also called extrinsic hemolytic anemia or autoimmune hemolytic anemia.* Drug-induced immune hemolytic anemia is rare; it can be mild or associated with severe hemolytic anemia and death. About 125 drugs have been implicated. Determining the drug causing the problem and stopping is the first step.[7]	• Cephalosporins • B-Lactam • NSAIDs • Methyldopa • Quinine/quinidine • Sulfa • Antineoplastics • Fludarabine
Macrocytic *Red blood cells are larger than normal with low levels of hemoglobin to carry oxygen; usually related to vitamin B12 or folate deficiency or malabsorption.* Causes of macrocytic anemia include myelodysplastic syndromes, bone marrow failure syndromes, aplastic anemia, plasma cell dyscrasia, alcoholic liver disease, myeloid malignancy, lymphoid cancer, chronic renal failure, solid tumors and vitamin B12 deficiency.[8]	• Antimetabolites • Chemotherapeutic agents • Dihydrofolate reductase inhibitors • Oral contraceptives • Anticonvulsants • Metformin
Sideroblastic *Inadequate marrow utilization of iron for heme synthesis despite the presence of adequate iron (iron utilization anemia). For both acquired and congenital sideroblastic anemia, heme synthesis is impaired.* Sideroblastic anemias (SAs) are anemias of disrupted iron utilization in the erythroblast with ineffective erythropoiesis and systemic iron overload. Acquired or congenital sideroblastic anemias require careful clinical and laboratory evaluation, including molecular analysis. Supportive treatments usually provide for a favorable prognosis and often for normal survival.[9]	• Chloramphenicol • Linezolid • Tetracycline • Busulfan • Isoniazid • Phenacetin • Progesterone
Red cell aplasia *PRCA is defined by a normocytic normochromic anemia with severe reticulocytopenia. There is significant reduction or absence of erythroid precursors from the bone marrow.* Primary acquired PRCA is an autoimmune disorder. Secondary acquired PRCA may be associated with collagen vascular/autoimmune disorders such as systemic lupus erythematosus; chronic lymphocytic leukemia or large granular lymphocyte leukemia; infections, particularly B19 parvovirus; thymoma and drugs; or toxic agents.[10]	• Carbamazepine • Valproic acid • ESAs • Sulfonamides • Chloramphenicol • Linezolid • Procainamide

Abbreviations: NSAIDs, nonsteroidal anti-inflammatory drugs; PRCA, pure red cell aplasia.
Data from Refs.[4,6–10]

by proinflammatory cytokines. Use of ESAs for the immediate correction of anemia is not recommended, as ESAs induce increase in reticulocytes after 72 to 96 hours.[1,13]

Substantial evidence, such decreased mortality and length of stay, to support broad use of ESAs in the ICU (except for specific indications such as renal disease or Jehovah's Witnesses), does not exist yet. Furthermore, considering the high doses of ESAs necessary to overcome inflammatory mediators in the critically ill, ESA therapy is also not economical.[1]

EMERGING EVIDENCE—MIXED RESULTS

In a recent meta-analysis of 9 randomized, controlled trials (RCTs) with 2607 critically ill trauma patients, the effect of ESAs was evaluated based on indications that ESAs may have beneficial effects beyond erythropoiesis, such as reduction in mortality rate. The glycoprotein that stimulates erythropoiesis may also exert neuroprotective and anti-inflammatory effects. A meta-analysis found that compared with placebo, ESAs were associated with significant reduction in mortality without an increase in the rate of lower limb proximal deep venous thrombosis. For patients with traumatic brain injury, the number of patients surviving with moderate disability or good recovery did not increase.[14] However, In another RCT examining neurologic recovery after traumatic brain injury, there was no survival benefit conferred with erythropoietin administration compared with placebo.[15]

Although anemia is obvious in trauma, for the patient with HF, anemia is often hidden. Many patients with systolic HF are placed on an angiotensin-converting enzyme inhibitor or an angiotensin receptor blocker, which provide morbidity and mortality benefits. Consider then the patient without HF; angiotensin II increases erythropoietin secretion by reducing renal blood flow through vasoconstrictive actions. When angiotensin-converting enzyme inhibitor or angiotensin receptor blocker therapy is used, erythropoietin secretion via this normal pathway does not occur. Other proposed causes of anemia in HF include proinflammatory cytokines, renal disease, and antiplatelet therapies.[13]

In a randomized, double-blind trial, 2278 patients with systolic HF and mild-to-moderate anemia (hemoglobin level, 9.0–12.0 g per deciliter) received either darbepoetin alfa (to achieve a hemoglobin target of 13 g per deciliter) or placebo. The primary outcomes were death from any cause or hospitalization for worsening HF. Treatment with darbepoetin alfa did not improve clinical outcomes in patients with systolic HF and mild-to-moderate anemia with use not supported in systolic HF.[16] Results should be interpreted considering the characteristics of the sample. The anemic patients enrolled in the RED-HF study were older, were moderately to markedly symptomatic, and had extensive comorbidity.[17]

A recent meta-analysis of evidence drawn from PubMed, Embase, Cochrane Central Register of Controlled Trials, and the US National Institutes of Health registry of clinical trials was completed to clarify the efficacy and safety of ESA use in HF. Thirteen RCTs were included in the analysis. Findings revealed that for HF patients with anemia, ESAs had a neutral effect on all-cause mortality and hospital readmission but improved dyspnea and quality of life. Although there was no specific increase in severe thromboembolic events, the overall risk for thromboembolic events increased with use.[18]

Reduction of symptom burden in HF with use of ESAs was also identified in another meta-analysis of 11 studies with 3044 patients. Again, no mortality benefit was identified. However, ESA therapy increased hemoglobin levels and ejection fraction, decreased B-type natriuretic protein, improved New York Heart Association functional class, and decreased hospitalizations.[19]

Evidence supporting use of ESAs to treat anemia in HF is promising but not conclusive. Although ESA therapy seems to improve hemoglobin, clinical outcomes related to exercise, and quality of life and reduces hospitalization, findings remain conflicting. Further research is needed to explain the relationship among anemia, symptom burden, and mortality in HF.[13] Low-quality evidence, small sample sizes, bias, and limited numbers of rigorous studies suggest keeping current with the literature with clinical judgment and knowledge of the patient in clinical management of anemia.[3]

The clinician needs to be mindful that off-label use of ESAs to treat anemia has safety concerns. In a meta-analysis of the safety of off-label use of ESAs in critically ill patients, results from 34 RCTs and 14 controlled observational studies in any language that compared off-label ESAs with other interventions, placebo, or no treatment were evaluated. Results showed that use of ESAs in the critically ill is associated with clinically relevant thrombotic vascular events.[12]

Therefore, "less may be more" when treating anemia in HF. The American College of Physicians recommends a restrictive posture in for red blood cell replacement with a treatment threshold of 7 to 8 g/dL. As for ESA use, patients with systolic HF may be the most appropriate group to benefit from therapy. For patients with mild-to-moderate anemia with congestive heart failure or coronary heart disease, the American College of Physicians recommends ESAs not to be prescribed, as harms seem to outweigh benefits particularly for thromboembolic events and possible increased risk for stroke. Additionally, iron therapy (intravenous iron) carboxymaltose in patients with New York Heart Association class III HF and low ferritin levels seem to provide short-term benefits such as increased exercise tolerance and quality of life. However, more evidence is needed, as possible harms and long-term outcomes of this therapy are unknown. Furthermore, further research of the risks and benefits of oral iron therapy in heart failure is needed.[3]

The Future

With increasing knowledge of the risks associated with receiving blood transfusions, a new paradigm of bloodless medicine is needed. Principles of bloodless medicine include careful monitoring for obvious and hidden anemias, rapid intervention, minimizing blood losses from laboratory testing and procedures, and careful management of bleeding diatheses. As evidence is revealed and refined, standard treatment of anemia in the ICU will include ESAs, iron, folate, and vitamin B12, which will reduce risks associated with blood transfusions.[20]

REFERENCES

1. Jelkmann I, Jelkmann W. Impact of erythropoietin on intensive care patients. Transfus Med Hemother 2013;40:310–8.
2. Corwin HL, Gettinger A, Pearl RG, et al. The CRIT study: anemia and blood transfusion in the critically ill- current clinical practice in the United States. Crit Care Med 2004;32(1):39–52.
3. Qaseem A, Humphrey L, Fitterman N, et al. Treatment of anemia in patients with heart disease: a clinical practice guideline from the American College of Physicians. Ann Intern Med 2013;159(11):770–9.
4. Shander A, Goodnough LT, Javidroozi M, et al. Iron deficiency anemia-bridging the knowledge and practice gap. Transfus Med Rev 2014;28(3):156–66.
5. Ngo K, Kotecha D, Walters JAE, et al. Erythropoiesis-stimulating agents for anaemia in chronic heart failure patients. Cochrane Database Syst Rev 2010;(1):CD007613.
6. Shander A, Javidroozi M, Ashton ME. Drug-induced anemia and other red cell disorders: a guide in the age of polypharmacy. Curr Clin Pharmacol 2011;6(4):295–303.
7. Garratty G. Immune hemolytic anemia associated with drug therapy. Blood Rev 2010;24(4–5):143–50.
8. Takahashi N, Kameoka J, Takahashi N, et al. Causes of macrocytic anemia among 628 patients: mean corpuscular volumes of 114 and 130 fL as critical markers for categorization. Int J Hematol 2016;104(3):344–57.

9. Bottomley SS, Fleming MD. Sideroblastic anemia: diagnosis and management. Hematol Oncol Clin North Am 2014;8(4):653–70.

10. Means RT. Pure red cell aplasia. Blood 2016;128(21):2504–9.

11. Hesdorffer C, Longo D. Drug-induced megaloblastic anemia. N Engl J Med 2015; 373(17):1649–58.

12. Mesgarpour B, Heidinger BH, Schwameis M, et al. Safety of off-label erythropoi-esis stimulating agents in critically ill patients: a meta-analysis. Intensive Care Med 2013;39(11):1896–908.

13. Lindquist DE, Cruz JL, Brown JN. Use of erythropoiesis-stimulating agents in the treatment of anemia in patients with systolic heart failure. J Cardiovasc Pharma-col Ther 2015;20(1):59–65.

14. French CJ, Glassford NJ, Gantner D, et al. Erythropoiesis-stimulating agents in critically Ill trauma patients: a systematic review and meta-analysis. Ann Surg 2017;265(1):54–62.

15. Robertson CS, Hannay HJ, Yamal JM, et al. Effect of erythropoietin and transfu-sion threshold on neurological recovery after traumatic brain injury: a randomized clinical trial. JAMA 2014;312(1):36–47.

16. Swedberg K, Young JB, Anand IS, et al. Treatment of anemia with darbepoetin alfa in systolic heart failure. N Engl J Med 2013;368(13):1210–9.

17. McMurray JJ, Anand IS, Diaz R, et al. Baseline characteristics of patients in the reduction of events with darbepoetin alfa in heart failure trial (RED-HF). Eur J Heart Fail 2013;15(3):334–41.

18. Kang J, Park J, Lee JM, et al. The effects of erythropoiesis stimulating therapy for anemia in chronic heart failure: a meta-analysis of randomized clinical trials. Int J Cardiol 2016;218:12–22.

19. Zhang H, Zhang P, Zhang Y, et al. Effects of erythropoiesis-stimulating agents on heart failure patients with anemia: a meta-analysis. Postepy Kardiol Interwencyj-nej 2016;12(3):247–53.

20. Resar L, Wick E, Almasri TN, et al. Bloodless medicine: current strategies and emerging treatment paradigms. Transfusion 2016;56(10):2637–47.

Use of High-Fidelity Simulation to Increase Knowledge and Skills in Caring for Patients Receiving Blood Products

Tonya Breymier, PhD, RN, CNE, COI[a],*,
Tonya Rutherford-Hemming, EdD, RN, ANP-BC, CHSE[b]

KEYWORDS

- High-fidelity simulation • Staff nurse development • Staff nurse competency
- Competency blood transfusions

KEY POINTS

- Simulation has evolved and has utility with staff development and staff nurse competency for blood transfusion management processes.
- Blood transfusion knowledge, skills, and practice can be simulated in a safe, learning environment.
- Simulation provides an environment to practice critical thinking and clinical judgment with blood transfusion management processes.
- Blood transfusion reactions do not occur frequently but high-fidelity simulation (HFS) provides practice and preparation for such situations.

INTRODUCTION

High-fidelity simulation (HFS) has emerged as a teaching technology with potential to increase knowledge and skills in caring for patients receiving blood products. This article describes the current state of the science related to the use of simulation in this critical life-saving skill. The history of simulation is discussed, along with a critique of the literature related to the use of simulation education for blood transfusion management competency in addition to a blood transfusion simulation example.

BACKGROUND
History of Simulation

Simulation is "a technique that creates a situation or environment to allow persons to experience a representation of a real event for the purpose of practice, learning,

[a] School of Nursing and Health Sciences, Indiana University East, 2325 Chester Boulevard, Richmond, IN 47374, USA; [b] School of Nursing, University of North Carolina-Greensboro, 408 Moore Building, P.O. Box 26170, Greensboro, NC 27402, USA
* Corresponding author.
E-mail address: tbreymie@iue.edu

Crit Care Nurs Clin N Am 29 (2017) 369–375
http://dx.doi.org/10.1016/j.cnc.2017.04.010
0899-5885/17/© 2017 Elsevier Inc. All rights reserved.

evaluation, testing, or to gain understanding of systems or human actions."[1] The history of simulation stretches back for centuries. The earliest use of simulation can be traced to the military, aviation, and nuclear power industries.[2] The military has used simulation the longest, dating back to the eighteenth century.[3] Aviation pioneered the modern use of simulation in the 1930s.[4] Simulation has been used because training or testing in these areas in the real world would be too dangerous or costly to undertake.

It was not until the second half of the twentieth century that medicine began using simulation.[2] Anesthesiology was the first area of medicine to embark on the use of clinical simulation.[5] Working with anesthetists, Laerdal developed the Resusci-Anne, a basic simulator that is still used today. The Resusci-Anne was a low-cost, effective part-task trainer that increased the effectiveness of resuscitation training.[2]

of Resusci-Anne came another form of simulation in medicine. The inception of the standardized patient was introduced by Barrows and Abrahamson[6] in 1963. According to Barrows,[7] the term standardized patient is, "the umbrella term for both a simulated patient (a well person trained to simulate a patient's illness in a standardized way) and an actual patient (who is trained to present his or her own illness in a standardized way)." Barrows saw the standardized patient as being able to provide students with additional training outside a textbook by putting them face to face with patients who could provide the physical, psychological, and emotional aspects of clinical practice.

Following the direction and development of Resusci-Anne, Sim One was developed in the late 1960s by Abrahamson and Denson.[3,8] Sim One was a manikin much like Resusci-Anne but more complex and sophisticated, having computer programs that elicited physiologic responses (breathing, heartbeat, pulses, blood pressure, blinking, and oxygen consumption).

Gordon[9] developed Harvey in the 1970s. This partial body simulator mimicked cardiac conditions and has been widely used since its invention. Then, in the late 1980s, Gaba and colleagues[10] resurrected the idea of HFS and developed models for use in the area of anesthesiology. This was the beginning of today's modern moderate to high-fidelity simulator that is commonly used for learning and training in the medical arena.

The influx of computer-based simulation emerged in the 1980s.[3,11] Computer-based simulations offered real-life scenarios that required appropriate user responses. Then, early in the twenty-first century, computer-based simulations progressed to virtual simulations.[3] In virtual simulations students can create self-figures, or avatars, to replicate a virtual life online and role play patient interaction scenarios. See **Table 1** for a summary of the history of simulation.

Table 1	
History of simulation	
Year	**Source**
1930s	Aviation
1960	Task trainers
1963	Standardized patients
1970s	Partial body simulators
1980s	HFSs & computer-based simulations
2000s	Virtual simulations

Major movements of the late twentieth century drove the impetus toward the use of simulation in the medical community. Changing clinical experiences, shorter times in training, and working time restrictions created skill deficiencies in medical students.[2,12] Simulation was implemented as an adjunct teaching methodology to counter the skill deficiencies.

In 1999, the Institute of Medicine (IOM)[13] published *To Err Is Human*, a report that brought patient safety issues to the forefront of health care and education. The report estimated that 45,000 to 98,000 patients die each year in the United States as a result of medical error. Based on this staggering number, the IOM called for systemic change in health care practices and argued that interdisciplinary training should be a top priority in educational institutions. The report highlighted the potential benefits of teamwork and identified simulation as a resource to address the needed reform.

USE OF SIMULATION FOR BLOOD TRANSFUSION MANAGEMENT COMPETENCY

According to the American Red Cross,[14] someone in the United States needs blood every 2 seconds, resulting in almost 21 million blood component transfusions each year. Nursing students rarely experience blood transfusion practices and protocols, let alone exposure to blood transfusion reactions. Despite the low incidence of transfusion reactions, practicing nurses must remain cognizant and competent concerning assessment and appropriate interventions of transfusion reactions. Blood transfusion has become a common practice in hospitals across the globe; safe practices and competency evaluation are paramount for reduced blood transfusion errors and safe patient care.

The literature is scarce regarding current competency training and evaluation of nurse's knowledge and skills with blood transfusion management and recognition of transfusion reactions. A descriptive study conducted in the United Kingdom found practicing nurses had knowledge deficits regarding blood transfusion practices.[15] A second study found that, even after specific training on safe transfusion practices, the participant's knowledge declined over time.[16] Factors such as work environment, workload, and distractions can have deleterious effects on safe transfusion practices.[17]

Quality improvement projects and evaluation studies supportive of the use of HFS for blood transfusion management competency are beginning to emerge in the literature. Campbell and colleagues[18] found blood transfusion simulation experiences with interdisciplinary teams identified areas for improvement and exposed safety issues with their current blood transfusion practices. Institutions must review and identify key elements in their current practices for safe blood transfusion management and include these elements within the simulation. **Box 1** outlines sample key elements for a simulated blood transfusion competency.

The International Association for Clinical Simulation and Learning (INACSL)[19] published *Standards of Best Practice: Simulation* in 2013, and updated it in 2015. The standards are free and accessible on the INACSL Web site. Rhees and colleagues[20] noted the importance of adequate before work, prebriefing, simulation design, and debriefing practices when using HFS for blood transfusion management competency. HFS can be a valuable education and competency evaluation experience,[21,22] but best practices and standards of simulation education should be followed for optimal outcomes.

Simulation Standards for Best Practice: Simulation

Specific steps to provide a quality HFS for blood transfusion management competency include

---

Box 1
Key elements for a simulated blood transfusion management competency

Patient chart review

Correct patient identification

Patient assessment, vital signs, and intravenous site patency

Follows institution policy and procedure for blood transfusion practices (eg, correct identification, two-person verification)

Assessment of blood transfusion reaction

Initiates appropriate nursing interventions based on patient reactions and assessment findings (eg, call physician, stop transfusion)

Therapeutic and professional communication

- HFS for blood transfusion simulation design
- Before work tutorial or lecture
- Prebriefing
- Simulation experience
- Debriefing.

It is important to identify the participant objectives for the simulation experience and ensure the participants are aware of the overall experience objectives. The simulation experience itself should be designed and reviewed by blood transfusion experts. INACSL *Standards for Best Practice: Simulation* standard IX: Design notes the institution should begin with a needs assessment to identify the overall outcome from the simulation experience.[23] It could be patient and blood product identification processes, pretransfusion and transfusion physical assessment procedures, and identification of transfusion reactions and appropriate nursing interventions, as well as post-transfusion assessment. Once objectives are identified from the needs assessment, then core content for a cognitive review should be planned. A before-work module can be created to outline the blood transfusion processes. The module can be delivered via face-to-face lecture or accessed online, depending on institution preference and time. **Table 2** outlines sample blood transfusion management simulation objectives and expected (learned) behaviors.

The blood transfusion process before-work module will be institution-specific, depending on institution policies and procedures for blood transfusions but could include similar topics contained in a teaching pack designed for nursing students.[21] The topic could include: whole blood testing, screening, and processing; sampling and patient selection; cross-matching; prescribing; pretransfusion assessment; bedside checking; initiating and monitoring the transfusion; and, post-transfusion assessment. A before-simulation lecture or before-work module can reduce the gap between education and practice, and offer a richer simulation and learning experience for the participant.[24] The before-work module will engage participants by including videos (ie, YouTube how-to videos) and/or gaming tutorials (https://www.nobelprize.org/educational/medicine/bloodtypinggame/).

Standards of Best Practice: Simulation standard IV: Facilitation[25] defines and identifies the importance of the prebriefing. This can vary from one simulation to the next but includes an orientation to the simulation environment, outlines facilitator and participant expectations, explains the roles of the participants, provides patient or experience background, and provides clear directions to the participants before the simulation experience. Because a manikin is used in HFS, orientation to the manikin is important, as well as the capabilities of the manikin and how physical

Table 2
Blood transfusion management simulation example

Simulation Objectives	Expected Behaviors
1. Identify patient risks in receiving blood products	Verbalized risks before simulation experience
2. Demonstrate correct procedure for blood product administration	• Complete assessment that includes vital signs and intravenous site evaluation for patency • Review chart for patient history, signed consent, physician orders, and pertinent laboratory values • Follow institution policy and protocol for blood administration procedure
3. Recognize signs and symptoms of a transfusion reaction	Recognize change in vital signs and/or patient complaints (eg, itching)
4. Use correct nursing interventions if patient experiences transfusion reaction	• Respond to patient complaints and/or signs and symptoms • Perform required actions related to patient complaints and/or signs and symptoms (ie, stop transfusion)
5. Practice appropriate therapeutic communication	Effective and therapeutic communication practiced throughout the simulation experience with patient, family members, and members of the health care team participating in the experience

assessment parameters will be assessed with the manikin. This same standard is applicable to the simulation facilitation itself. The facilitator needs to be experienced in simulation and understand that the simulation needs to play out the predetermined time frame. A list of participant expectations and behaviors may prove helpful for evaluation and providing cues (either from the facilitator or HFS manikin) to assist the participant to meet the desired experience outcomes. **Table 3** offers a generic

Table 3
Sample simulation template

Simulation Scenario			
Disciplines	Simulation Date		
Simulation objectives	Assigned simulation before work (must be completed before simulation experience)		
Prebriefing: Orientation to simulation laboratory or center, orientation to manikin, orientation to simulation supplies, patient chart, and so forth			
Patient history	Admitting diagnosis Allergies		
Significant laboratory values	Medical orders		
Equipment needed (include relevant settings)	Supplies needed		
Simulation Algorithm			
Time frame	Manikin reactions	Participant interventions	Cues from facilitators
0–5 min			
6–10 min			
11–17 min			
18–20 min			
References used to support simulation			

simulation template that could be used for a blood transfusion management simulation experience.

On completion of the simulation experience, the participants should be debriefed. The INACSL *Standards of Best Practice: Simulation* standard VI: The Debriefing Process outlines best practices for appropriate debriefing. The foundation for optimal debriefing is conducting the debriefing in a safe environment, providing confidentiality, and the facilitator should be experienced in debriefings, as well as the facilitator or observer of the simulation.[26] A good debriefing will follow a structured debriefing model and provide an avenue for open communication, trust, and reflection for improved future practices.

SUMMARY

HFS for blood transfusion management competency can provide a safe and valuable learning experience for staff nurses, in addition to providing a platform for interprofessional education (IPE).[20] Using HFS for blood transfusion management competency, as well as IPE, can create a learning experience that promotes team-based care and opportunities for participants to understand each discipline's unique role and responsibilities with blood transfusion management.[18]

As simulation education continues to grow within health education programs, there will undoubtedly be more and more competency training and evaluation using simulation. It is paramount for institutions to follow *Standards of Best Practice: Simulation*, in addition to providing staff development professionals and educators the tools, training, and resources to offer quality simulations based on best practices for simulation education.

REFERENCES

1. Lopreiato JO, editor. Downing D, Gammon W, et al, the Terminology & Concepts Working Group. Healthcare Simulation DictionaryTM. 2016. Available at: http://www.ssih.org/dictionary. Accessed January 3, 2017.
2. Bradley P. The history of simulation in medical education and possible future directions. Med Educ 2006;40:254–62.
3. Singh H, Kalani M, Acosta-Torres S, et al. History of simulation in medicine: from Resusci Annie to the Ann Myers Medical Center. Neurosurgery 2013;73(4):S9–14.
4. The National Center for Simulation. Early history of flight simulation. 2016. Available at: https://www.simulationinformation.com/education/early-history-flight-simulation. Accessed January 3, 2017.
5. Sinz EH. Anesthesiology national CME program and ASA activities in simulation. Anesthesiol Clin 2007;25:209–23.
6. Barrows HS, Abrahamson S. The programmed patient: a technique for appraising student performance in clinical neurology. J Med Educ 1964;39:802–5.
7. Barrows HS. An overview of the uses of standardized patients for teaching and evaluating clinical skills. Acad Med 1993;68(6):443–51.
8. Abrahamson S. Sim one–A patient simulator ahead of its time. Caduceus 1997;13(2):29–41.
9. Gordon MS. Cardiology patient simulator: development of an automated manikin to teach cardiovascular disease. Am J Cardiol 1974;34:350–5.
10. Aggarwal R, Mytton OT, Derbrew M, et al. Training and simulation for patient safety. Qual Saf Health Care 2010;19(Suppl 2):i34–43.

11. Fukui Y, Smith NT. Interactions among ventilation, the circulation and the uptake and distribution of halothane-use of a hybrid computer multiple model, I: the basic model. Anesthesiology 1981;54(2):107–18.

12. Issenberg SB, McGaghie WC, Petrusa ER, et al. Features and uses of high-fidelity medical simulations that lead to effective learning: a BEME systematic review. Med Teach 2005;27(1):10–28.

13. Kohn L, Corrigan J, Donaldson M, editors. To err is human: building a safer health system. Committee on quality of health care in America, Institute of Medicine. Washington, DC: National Academy Press; 1999.

14. American Red Cross. Blood facts and statistics. 2016. Available at: http://www.redcrossblood.org/learn-about-blood/blood-facts-and-statistics. Accessed January 3, 2017.

15. Hijji B, Parahoo K, Hussein MM, et al. Knowledge of blood transfusion among nurses. J Clin Nurs 2012;22:2536–50.

16. Smith A, Gray A, Atherton I, et al. Does time matter? An investigation of knowledge and attitudes following blood transfusion training. Nurse Educ Pract 2013;14(2):176–82.

17. Heddle NM, Fung M, Hervig T, et al. Challenges and opportunities to prevent transfusion errors: a qualitative evaluation for safer transfusion (QUEST). Transfusion 2012;52:1687–95.

18. Campbell DM, Poost-Foroosh L, Pavenski K, et al. Simulation as a toolkit: understanding the perils of blood transfusion in a complex health care environment. Adv Simulation 2016;1(32):1–10.

19. International Nursing Association for Clinical Simulation and Learning. Standards of best practice: simulation SM. 2016. Available at: http://www.inacsl.org/i4a/pages/index.cfm?pageid=3407. Accessed October 23, 2016.

20. Rhees JR, Scheese CH, Ward D, et al. Clinical practice simulation for blood transfusion reactions: an interprofessional approach. Clin Lab Sci 2015;28(4):224–31.

21. Mole LJ, Hogg G, Benvie S. Evaluation of a teaching pack designed for nursing students to acquire the essential knowledge for competent practice in blood transfusion administration. Nurse Education Pract 2007;7:228–37.

22. Prentice D, O'Rourke T. Safe practice: using high-fidelity simulation to teach blood transfusion reactions. J Infus Nurs 2013;36(3):207–10.

23. Lioce L, Meakim CH, Fey MK, et al. Standards of best practice: simulation standard IX: simulation design. Clin Simulation Nurs 2015;11(6):309–15.

24. Flood L, Higbie J. A comparative assessment of nursing students' cognitive knowledge of blood transfusion using lecture and simulation. Nurse Educ Pract 2016;16:8–13.

25. Franklin AE, Boese T, Gloe D, et al. Standards of best practice: simulation standard IV: facilitation. Clin Simulation Nurs 2013;9(6S):S19–21.

26. Decker S, Fey M, Sideras S, et al. Standards of best practice: simulation standard VI: the debriefing process. Clin Simulation Nurs 2013;9(6S):S27–9.

Resources for Hematology On and Off the Web

Shirley Sebald-Kinder, MLS, AHIP[a], Janet L. Petty, MLIS, AHIP[b],*

KEYWORDS

- Evidence-based practice • Grading scales • Hematology • PICO
- Patient education • Consumer health

KEY POINTS

- The expansion of information, although improving patient outcomes, is hard to keep up with in health care.
- Evidence-based practice has developed as a way to filter out unreliable, low-quality information by providing steps for critically analyzing and grading the information to provide best-practice care.
- Resources for hematology-related information include journal articles, books, databases, and organizations.
- Locating hematology information for patients and family members is one of the most challenging of all health care topics.

INTRODUCTION

According to some estimations, medical information has been doubling every 5 years since 2000.[1] Consequently, as technology continues to advance, allowing easier access to the Internet, it has created a worldwide information "explosion." This process has contributed to improved patient outcomes because health care information used to diagnose and treat patients is now accessible at the point of care for health care providers.

Physicians currently need to read 7287 articles per month or 29 hours per week to keep up with published literature in the primary care field.[2] McGrath and colleagues[3] projected that more than 500,000 articles would be added to the health care literature during 2012. Evidence-based practice has emerged as the standard for providing quantifiable, reliable clinical care outcomes with randomized controlled trials, systematic reviews, meta-analyses, and clinical practice guidelines.[4–6]

[a] Premier Health Learning Institute, Craig Memorial Library, Miami Valley Hospital, One Wyoming Street, Dayton, OH 45409, USA; [b] Patient and Family Education, Premier Health Learning Institute, Craig Memorial Library, Miami Valley Hospital, One Wyoming Street, Dayton, OH 45409, USA
* Corresponding author.
E-mail address: jlpetty@premierhealth.com

Crit Care Nurs Clin N Am 29 (2017) 377–387
http://dx.doi.org/10.1016/j.cnc.2017.04.006
ccnursing.theclinics.com

Accrediting and certification bodies continue to drive standards, ensuring clinicians have access to knowledge-based information resources. The Joint Commission guidelines state that information should be accessible 24 hours a day, 7 days a week.[7] In addition, nursing research and evidence-based practice is a key part of the American Nurses Credentialing Center's Magnet model for new knowledge, innovations and improvements.[8]

EVIDENCE-BASED PRACTICE

The nursing literature database, Cumulative Index to Nursing and Allied Health Literature (CINAHL), contains 4.8 million citations[9] and the US National Library of Medicine database, PubMed, includes more than 22 million citations and abstracts.[10] The ability to navigate through information from books, journals, point-of-care products, and organizational Web sites presents multiple challenges to health care providers to keep abreast of new technologies and approaches to patient care. Furthermore, evidence-based practice involves multiple elements: (1) the use of current patient-centered research that has been determined to provide the best patient outcomes; (2) the clinician's expertise; and (3) the patient's specific values, preferences, and needs.[4,6] In order to provide information that is research-based/evidence-based; current; reliable; high quality; and, most important, safe for the patient, information should meet certain requirements, which include the following.

Before searching the literature, the question must first be formulated into the PICO(T) format, which helps clinicians focus on the population/patient/problem being studied, intervention to be used, comparison of the intervention, outcomes and, if needed, time factors. The PICO(T) format assists when questioning cause, diagnosis, therapy, prognosis, and prevention.[11] The following example is one approach using PICO(T) related to cause. Are type 2 diabetic patients (P), who take metformin (I), compared with type 2 diabetics who do not take metformin (C), at a greater risk for developing vitamin B_{12} deficiency (O) over a period of 1 year (T)?[12,13]

The next step is to search the literature using evidence-based databases (Cochrane Library, Joanna Briggs Institute), guidelines (National Guideline Clearinghouse), point-of-care tools (DynaMed, UpToDate), journal databases (CINAHL, PubMed), and organizations (National Hemophilia Foundation, Centers for Disease Control and Prevention). Another reliable resource providing lists of evidence-based resources is Essential Nursing Resources from the Interagency Council on Information Resources in Nursing.[14]

Once a search of the literature is completed, it is then important to appraise the literature critically to determine whether the information obtained answers the PICO(T) question. Carefully examine the results, validity, and reliability of the studies, as well as benefits to the patient when using this practice. Important factors to evaluate include when the study was completed, the date that the results of the study were published, investigators' credentials, any endorsements by governing bodies or organizations, type of patients studied, type of research (randomized, observational), and how the evidence was graded.[15–17]

Specific grading scales can be used when evaluating the literature, such as Joanna Briggs Institute, Grading of Recommendations, Assessment, Development and Evaluation (GRADE), Agency for Healthcare Research and Quality (AHRQ), or the United States Task Force on Community Preventive Services. The levels of recommendations vary depending on the grading scale used to evaluate the literature. Recommendations can be strong; moderate; sufficient; expert opinion; or not supported, being insufficient under research design, consistency of results, number of studies, or effectiveness.[18–20]

GRADING SCALES

Joanna Briggs Institute. The JBI Approach[21]: www.joannabriggs.org/jbi-approach. html

GRADE. GRADE Handbook[22]: www.gradeworkinggroup.org

AHRQ Methods Guide for Comparative Effectiveness Reviews. Grading the strength of a body of evidence when assessing health care interventions for the Effective Health Care Program of the Agency for Healthcare Research and Quality: an update[23]: https://effectivehealthcare.ahrq.gov/search-for-guides-reviews-and-reports/?pageaction=d

United States Preventive Services Task Force. The guide to clinical preventive services, 2014[24]: www.uspreventiveservicestaskforce.org

To read or print this guide, click on "Information for Health Professionals" and click on the document.

PROFESSIONAL HEMATOLOGY RESOURCES

When looking for information related to hematology issues in critical care, several resources are available on the Internet. Some of the databases are available primarily in libraries, whereas others allow free access to information via the Internet. No matter what resource is used, remember to perform a critical analysis of the information to determine whether the information meets your needs for providing sound, evidence-based clinical decisions.

Begin your search by discovering what information is available in the primary literature found in CINAHL, PubMed, and ClinicalKey for Nursing. For evidence-based reviews, the Cochrane Library includes the Database of Abstracts of Reviews of Effects (DARE) and Cochrane Database of Systematic Reviews. The Joanna Briggs Institute provides evidence-based systematic reviews, evidence summaries, and clinical guidelines. Others are aggregators of information, such as ACCESSSS Federated Search, which includes Nursing+ from McMaster University. ACCESSSS Federated Search and Nursing+ searches for topics across PubMed, Plus Studies, ACP Journal Club, Cochrane's DARE, EBM Guidelines, DynaMed, and UpToDate. DynaMed includes several evidence-based hematology topics, such as hematopoietic stem cell transplantation, plasma cell neoplasms, red blood cell disorders, white blood cell disorders, and transfusion medicine. UpToDate also includes hematology topics, including treatment of iron deficiency anemia in adults, indications and hemoglobin thresholds for red blood cell transfusion in adults, and clinical and laboratory aspects of platelet transfusion therapy. Organization and government Web sites have a wealth of information, and a few of these sources are mentioned later, as well as books and journals.

DATABASES

Accessed December 12, 2016

ACCESSSS Federated Search and Nursing+
McMaster University, Hamilton, Ontario, Canada
https://plus.mcmaster.ca/ACCESSSS/Default.aspx?Page=1
Subscription required for certain areas of the database

CINAHL
EBSCO Information Services, Ipswich, Massachusetts
www.ebscohost.com
Subscription required

ClinicalKey for Nursing
  Elsevier
  www.clinicalkey.com
  Subscription required
DynaMed Plus
  EBSCO, Ipswich, Massachusetts
  www.dynamed.com
  Subscription required
EBM Guidelines
  John Wiley and Sons, Inc
  http://onlinelibrary.wiley.com/book/10.1002/0470057203
  Subscription required
Essential Nursing Resources
  Interagency Council on Information Resources in Nursing
  http://www.icirn.org/Homepage/Essential-Nursing-Resources/default.aspx
  Free
Joanna Briggs Institute
  Joanna Briggs Institute, University of Adelaide, South Australia, Australia
  www.joannabriggs.org
  Subscription required
Lippincott Procedures
  Wolters Kluwer
  http://lippincottsolutions.com
  Subscription required
PubMed
  National Center for Biotechnology Information, National Library of Medicine, Na-
    tional Institutes of Health, Bethesda, Maryland
  www.ncbi.nlm.nih.gov/pubmed
  Free
UpToDate
  Wolters Kluwer
  www.uptodate.com
  Subscription required

ORGANIZATIONS

Accessed December 12, 2016
  American Association of Blood Banks
    www.aabb.org
    Free, and membership allows access to other resources
  American Association of Critical Care Nurses
    www.aacn.org/
  American Red Cross
    www.redcross.org
  American Society of Hematology: Image Bank
    www.hematology.org
  US Centers for Disease Control and Prevention: Blood Safety
    www.cdc.gov/bloodsafety/index.html
  US Food and Drug Administration: Blood and Blood Products
    http://www.fda.gov/BiologicsBloodVaccines/BloodBloodProducts/
  National Guideline Clearinghouse: AHRQ
    www.guideline.gov

National Institute for Health and Care Excellence
www.nice.org.uk/
National Hemophilia Foundation: Blood Safety
www.hemophilia.org/Bleeding-Disorders/Blood-Safety
World Health Organization
www.who.int

JOURNALS

Collins S, MacIntyre C, Hewer I. Thromboelastography: clinical application, interpretation, and transfusion management. AANA J 2016;84:129–34.

Daru J, Cooper NA, Khan KS. Systematic review of randomized trials of the effect of iron supplementation on iron stores and oxygen carrying capacity in pregnancy. Acta Obstet Gynecol Scand 2016;95:270–9.

Du Y, Ye M, Zheng F. Active management of the third stage of labor with and without controlled cord traction: a systematic review and meta-analysis of randomized controlled trials. Acta Obstet Gynecol Scand 2014;93:626–33.

Peyrin-Biroulet L, Williet N, Cacoub P. Guidelines on the diagnosis and treatment of iron deficiency across indications: a systematic review. Am J Clin Nutr 2015;102:1585–94.

Muñoz M, Gómez-Ramírez S, Kozek-Langeneker S. Pre-operative haematological assessment in patients scheduled for major surgery. Anaesthesia 2016;71(Suppl 1):19–28.

Kaufman RM, Djulbegovic B, Gernsheimer T, et al. Platelet transfusion: a clinical practice guideline from the AABB. Ann Intern Med 2015;162:205–13.

Chan AW, de Gara CJ. An evidence-based approach to red blood cell transfusions in asymptomatically anaemic patients. Ann R Coll Eng 2015;97:556–62.

Mavros MN, Xu L, Maqsood H, et al. Perioperative blood transfusion and the prognosis of pancreatic cancer surgery: systematic review and meta-analysis. Ann Surg Oncol 2015;22:4382–91.

Alexander PE, Barty R, Fei Y, et al. Transfusion of fresher vs older red blood cells in hospitalized patients: a systematic review and meta-analysis. Blood 2016;127:400–10.

Docherty AB, O'Donnell R, Brunskill S, et al. Effect of restrictive versus liberal transfusion strategies on outcomes in patients with cardiovascular disease in a non-cardiac surgery setting: systematic review and meta-analysis. BMJ 2016;352:i1351.

Holst LB, Petersen MW, Haase N, et al. Restrictive versus liberal transfusion strategy for red blood cell transfusion: systematic review of randomized trials with meta-analysis and trial sequential analysis. BMJ 2015;350:h1354.

Qian C, Wei B, Ding J, et al. The efficacy and safety of iron supplementation in patients with heart failure and iron deficiency: a systematic review and meta-analysis. Can J Cardiol 2016;32:151–9.

Da Luz LT, Nascimento B, Shankarakutty AK, et al. Effect of thromboelastography (TEG®) and rotational thromboelastometry (ROTEM®) on diagnosis of coagulopathy, transfusion guidance and mortality in trauma: description systematic review. Crit Care 2014;18:518.

Mirski MA, Frank SM, Kor DJ, et al. Restrictive and liberal red cell transfusion strategies in adult patients: reconciling clinical data with best practice. Crit Care 2015;19:202.

Giralt S, Garderet L, Durie B, et al. American Society of Blood and Marrow Transplantation, European Society of Blood and Marrow Transplantation, Blood and Marrow Transplant Clinical Trials Network, and International Myeloma Working Group Consensus Conference on Salvage Hematopoietic Cell Transplantation in Patients with Relapsed Multiple Myeloma. Biol Blood Marrow Transplant 2015;21:2039–51.

Majhail NS, Farnia SH, Carpenter PA, et al. Indications for autologous and allogeneic hematopoietic cell transplantation: guidelines from the American Society for Blood and Marrow Transplantation. Biol Blood Marrow Transplant 2015;21:1863–9.

Peffault de Latour R, Peters C, Gibson B, et al. Recommendations on hematopoietic stem cell transplantation for inherited bone marrow failure syndromes. Bone Marrow Transplant 2015;50:1168–72.

Hough R, Danby R, Russell N, et al. Recommendations for standard UK approach to incorporating umbilical cord blood into clinical transplantation practice: an update on cord blood unit selection, donor selection algorithms and conditioning protocols. Br J Haematol 2016;172:360–70.

Killick SB, Bown N, Cavenagh J, et al. Guidelines for the diagnosis and management of adult aplastic anaemia. Br J Haematol 2016;172:187–207.

Motta M, Del Vecchio A, Chirico G. Fresh frozen plasma administration in the neonatal intensive care unit: evidence-based guidelines. Clin Perinatol 2015;42:639–50.

Nadisauskiene RJ, Kliucinskas M, Dobozinskas P, et al. The impact of postpartum haemorrhage management guidelines implemented in clinical practice: a systematic review of the literature. Eur J Obstet Gynecol Reprod Biol 2014;178:21–6.

Ng MS, Ng AS, Chan J, et al. Effects of packed red blood cell storage duration on post-transfusion clinical outcomes: a meta-analysis and systematic review. Intensive Care Med 2015;41:2087–97.

Menendez JB, Edwards B. Early identification of acute hemolytic transfusion reactions: realistic implications for best practice in patient monitoring. Medsurg Nurs 2016;25:88–90, 109.

Backes CH, Rivera BK, Haque U, et al. Placental transfusion strategies in very preterm neonates: a systematic review and meta-analysis. Obstet Gynecol 2014;124:47–56.

Teng Z, Zhu Y, Liu Y, et al. Restrictive blood transfusion strategies and associated infection in orthopedic patients: a meta-analysis of 8 randomized controlled trials. Sci Rep 2015;5:13421.

Elhenawy AM, Meyer SR, Bagshaw SM, et al. Role of preoperative intravenous iron therapy to correct anemia before major surgery: study protocol for systematic review and meta-analysis. Syst Rev 2015;4:29.

Abdul-Kadir R, McLintock C, Ducloy AS, et al. Evaluation and management of postpartum hemorrhage: consensus from an international expert panel. Transfusion 2014;54:1756–68.

Kumar A, Mhaskar R, Grossman BJ, et al. Platelet transfusion: a systematic review of the clinical evidence. Transfusion 2015;55:1116–27.

McQuilten ZK, Crighton G, Engelbrecht S, et al. Transfusion interventions in critical bleeding requiring massive transfusion: a systematic review. Transfus Med Rev 2015;29:127–37.

Ludwig H, Evstatiev R, Kornek G, et al. Iron metabolism and iron supplementation in cancer patients. Wien Klin Wochenschr 2015;127:907–19.

BOOKS

Baggott C. Anemia. In: Kline NE, editor. Essentials of pediatric hematology/oncology nursing: a core curriculum. 4th edition. Chicago (IL): Association of Pediatric Hematology/Oncology Nurses; 2014. p. 92–5.

Bain BJ, Bates I, Laffan MA, et al. Dacie and Lewis practical haematology. 11th edition. Edinburgh: Elsevier Churchill Livingstone; 2012.

DeLoughery TG, editor. Hemostasis and thrombosis, 3rd edition. New York: Springer; 2015.

Desrosiers KP, Corwin HL. Anemia and red blood cell transfusion in critically ill patients. In: Hall JB, Schmidt GA, Kress JP, editors. Principles of critical care. 4th edition. New York: McGraw-Hill Education; 2015. p. 842–4.

Dressler DK. Hematologic and immune systems. In: Burns SM, editor. AACN Essentials of critical care nursing. 3rd edition. New York: McGraw-Hill Education/Medical; 2014. p. 337–49.

Glaspy J. Disorders of blood cell production in clinical oncology. In: Niederhuber JE, Armitage JO, Doroshow JH, et al, editors. Abeloff's clinical oncology. 5th edition. Philadelphia: Elsevier Saunders; 2014. p. 532–41.

Greer JP, List AF, Rodgers GM, et al, editors. Wintrobe's clinical hematology. 13th edition. Philadelphia: Wolters Kluwer/Lippincott Williams & Wilkins; 2014.

Hoffman R, Benz EJ Jr, Silberstein LE, et al. Hematology: basic principles and practice. 6th edition. Philadelphia: Elsevier Saunders; 2013.

Jaffe ES, Vardiman J. WHO classification of hematologic malignancies. In: Niederhuber JE, Armitage JO, Doroshow JH, et al, editors. Abeloff's clinical oncology. 5th edition. Philadelphia: Elsevier Saunders; 2014. p. 219–25.

Jones MP, Arbo JE. Transfusion therapy. In: Arbo JE, Ruoss SJ, Lighthall GK, et al, editors. Decision making in emergency critical care: an evidence-based handbook. Philadelphia: Wolters Kluwer; 2015. p. 387–93.

Kaushansky K, Lichtman MA, Prchal JT, et al. Williams hematology. 9th edition. New York: McGraw-Hill Education; 2016.

Lachant NA. Hemorrhagic and thrombotic disorders. In: Parrillo JE, Dellinger RP, editors. Critical care medicine: principles of diagnosis and management in the adult. 4th edition. Philadelphia: Elsevier Saunders; 2014. p. 1363–75.

Hematology and oncology. In: Merck manual professional version. Kenilworth (NJ); 2016. Available at: www.merckmanuals.com/professional/hematology-and-oncology. Accessed September 10, 2016.

Marik PE. Transfusion of blood and blood products. In: Evidence-based critical care. 3rd edition. New York: Springer; 2015. p. 585–619.

Marino PL. Disorders of circulatory flow. In: Marino's The ICU book. 4th edition. Philadelphia: Wolters Kluwer/Lippincott Williams and Wilkins; 2014. p. 195–282.

Marino PL. Blood components. In: Marino's The ICU book. 4th edition. Philadelphia: Wolters Kluwer/Lippincott Williams and Wilkins; 2014. p. 349–90.

Orkin SH, Fisher DE, Ginsburg D, et al. Nathan and Oski's hematology and oncology of infancy and childhood. 8th edition. Philadelphia: Elsevier Saunders; 2015.

Shen MC, Zimmerman JL. Use of blood components in the intensive care unit. In: Parrillo JE, Dellinger RP, editors. Critical care medicine: principles of diagnosis and management in the adult. 4th edition. Philadelphia: Elsevier Saunders; 2014. p. 1376–93.

Thomas K. Bleeding disorders. In: Hall JB, Schmidt GA, Kress JP, editors. Principles of critical care. 4th edition. New York: McGraw-Hill Education; 2015. p. 844–57.

CONSUMER HEALTH HEMATOLOGY RESOURCES

Locating hematology information for patient and family members is challenging. Hematology can be technical and difficult for most people to understand, especially for those with little or no science background and poor reading skills. In addition, many hematologic conditions are not addressed in consumer or lay language resources, which then requires clinicians to present difficult material in language the patients can understand and then act on appropriately. There is even less information available in languages other than English and Spanish. Although there are vendors that provide online patient education materials, for common health conditions and medications, there remains a lack of resources on a wide variety of hematologic conditions.

Providing health information that patients can understand is not only a requirement but also necessary for patients to make changes to improve their health outcomes, if they so choose. The following are resources (not exhaustive) that provide credible, lay language (consumer health/patient education) information on various hematologic conditions. Although these are geared to the patient, the reading level is still high because of the subject matter and is likely to be difficult for poor readers to understand without assistance from the health care provider.

American Society for Blood and Marrow Transplantation
asbmt.org/
    Once at this site click on "Patient Education" to find information on terms and definitions, including information on several blood disorders, umbilical cord blood storage, and external resources that link to many groups offering education and support for blood and bone marrow transplantation patients.

Aplastic Anemia and MDS International Foundation
www.aamds.org/
    This site is devoted to patients with bone marrow failure disease and provides information on diseases affecting the bone marrow, treatments, and support resources.

BE THE MATCH
www.bethematch.org/
    This site provides information covering transplant basics, patient stories, resources that explain a variety of blood disorders, their treatment, and support. This site provides print resources in several languages, and provides support by phone in more than 100 languages.

The Bone Marrow Foundation
www.bonemarrow.org/
    Once at this site, click on "Resources for Patients and Families" to find many resources, including 2 booklets on allogeneic and autologous transplantation (both available in English and Spanish).

ConsumerHealthChoices
www.consumerhealthchoices.org/
    ConsumerHealthChoices is where free Consumer Reports resources for patients and families can be found. Once at the site, click on "Patients and Families" to obtain a handout called *Blood Transfusions for Anemia in the Hospital*, which is available in English and Spanish.

KidsHealth
  www.kidshealth.org/
    KidsHealth provides information written in plain language on a wide range of health issues, including blood disorders, transfusions, and medical tests geared to parents, teens, and children.

Leukemia and Lymphoma Society
  www.lls.org/
    Once at this site, click on "Patients and Caregivers" to find extensive resources on disease information, education (booklets available to download), and support resources. This site may also be viewed in Spanish, Canadian English, and French Canadian.

Merck Manual Consumer Version
  www.merckmanuals.com/home
    This site provides excellent resources on several blood disorders, such as anemias, bleeding caused by abnormal blood vessels, bleeding caused by clotting disorders, as well as a basic overview of the biology of blood. The site also provides resources on pronunciations, medical terms, common medical tests, images, audio, video, and many others. In addition to English, 8 other languages are available to the reader.

National Hemophilia Foundation for all bleeding disorders
  www.hemophilia.org/
    This site provides a wide variety of information on bleeding disorders, inhibitors and other complications, blood safety, future therapies, and a link to Steps for Living, which provides information for all ages from birth to adult with a bleeding disorder. Steps for Living is also available in Spanish.

Patient
  www.patient.info/
    This Web site from the United Kingdom is accredited by The Information Standard, NHS England's quality mark. This site has a wide range of health topics written for patients and includes blood disorders. In addition, this site provides PatientPlus articles that are written by UK doctors and based on research evidence and UK and European guidelines geared to health professionals.

WebMD
  www.webmd.com/
    Although this site is filled with advertisements it provides a broad range of topics on blood and blood disorders written for consumers.

X-Plain Patient Education
  www.patient-education.com/patients.html
    A variety of patient education information is available in print and in an audiovisual format that is available in English, Spanish, and Arabic.

SUMMARY

At times, searching the literature can be challenging because of the large volume of information now available. Obtaining evidence can be time consuming to locate and determine what is valid and reliable, and which evidence will drive the best patient outcomes. Studies have shown that many nurses do not have the time, the access to knowledge-based resources, or expertise to find evidence. However, librarians do have the knowledge and skills to provide expert searching strategies using databases, such as CINAHL, PubMed, Cochrane Library, and so forth.[25] Librarians are valuable members of the health care team that can save clinicians time while supporting clinical decisions leading to improved patient outcomes.[26] The rapid expansion of medical information, even though clinicians have greater access, does not decrease the need for librarian-mediated searching. The knowledge information explosion has increased the need to seek assistance from a professional health sciences librarian who will gladly provide this expertise and assistance.

REFERENCES

1. Mattox DE. Welcome to archives CME. Arch Otolaryngol Head Neck Surg 2000; 126:914.
2. Alper BS, Hand JA, Elliott SG, et al. How much effort is needed to keep up with the literature relevant for primary care? J Med Libr Assoc 2004;92:429–37.
3. McGrath JM, Brown RE, Samra HA. Before you search the literature: how to prepare and get the most out of citation databases. Newborn Infant Nurs Rev 2012; 12:162–70.
4. Straus SE, Glasziou P, Richardson WS, et al. Introduction. Evidence-based medicine: how to practice and teach it. 4th edition. New York: Churchill Livingstone Elsevier; 2011. p. 1–12.
5. Rebar CR, Gersch CJ. Evidence-based healthcare: using research in practice. In: Rebar CR, Gersch CJ, editors. Understanding research for evidence-based practice. 4th edition. Philadelphia: Wolters Kluwer; 2015. p. 1–26.
6. Melnyk BM, Fineout-Overholt E. Making the case for evidence-based practice and cultivating a spirit of inquiry. In: Melnyk BM, Fineout-Overholt E, editors. Evidence-based practice in nursing & health care: a guide to best practice. 3rd edition. Philadelphia: Wolters Kluwer; 2015. p. 3–23.
7. Information management. The Joint Commission. Comprehensive Accreditation Manual Hospitals. Oak Brook (IL): Joint Commission Resources; 2016. Available at: https://e-dition.jcrinc.com/MainContent.aspx. Accessed October 6, 2016.
8. American Nurses Credentialing Center. Announcing a new model for ANCC's magnet recognition program©. Silver Spring (MD): American Nurses Credentialing Center. Magnet News; 2008. Available at: http://www.nursecredentialing.org/Magnet/MagnetNews/2008-MagnetNews/NewMagnetModel.html. Accessed December 21, 2016.
9. CINAHL Plus with Full Text: Full-text nursing and allied health literature plus additional resources. 2016. Available at: https://health.ebsco.com/products/cinahl-plus-with-full-text. Accessed October 1, 2016.
10. Canese K, Weis S. PubMed: the bibliographic database. 2013. Available at: https://www.ncbi.nlm.nih.gov/books/NBK153385/?report=printable. Accessed October 1, 2016.
11. Stillwell SB, Fineout-Overholt E, Melnyk BM, et al. Evidence-based practice step by step: asking the clinical question: a key step in evidence-based practice. Am J Nurs 2010;110:58–61.
12. Langan RC, Zawistoski KJ. Update on vitamin B_{12} deficiency. Am Fam Physician 2011;83:1425–30.
13. Fineout-Overholt E, Stillwell SB. Asking compelling, clinical questions. In: Melnyk BM, Fineout-Overholt E, editors. Evidence-based practice in nursing & healthcare: a guide to best practice. 3rd edition. Philadelphia: Wolters Kluwer; 2015. p. 24–39.

14. Schnall JG, Fowler S. Essential nursing resources. 26th edition. Silver Spring (MD): Interagency Council on Information Resources in Nursing; 2012. Available at: http://www.icirn.org/Homepage/Essential-Nursing-Resources/default.aspx. Accessed October 24, 2016.
15. LoBiondo-Wood G. Systematic reviews and clinical practice guidelines. In: LoBiondo-Wood G, Haber J, editors. Nursing research: methods and critical appraisal for evidence-based practice. 8th edition. St Louis (MO): Elsevier Mosby; 2014. p. 218–30.
16. Fulton S, Krainovich-Miller B. Gathering and appraising the literature. In: LoBiondo-Wood G, Haber J, editors. Nursing research: methods and critical appraisal for evidence-based practice. 8th edition. St Louis (MO): Elsevier Mosby; 2014. p. 49–74.
17. Fineout-Overholt E, Melnyk BM, Stillwell SB, et al. Evidence-based practice step by step: critical appraisal of the evidence: part II. Am J Nurs 2010;110:41–8.
18. Titler M. Developing an evidence-based practice. In: LoBiondo-Wood G, Haber J, editors. Nursing research: methods and critical appraisal for evidence-based practice. 8th edition. St Louis (MO): Elsevier Mosby; 2014. p. 418–41.
19. Kavanagh BP. The GRADE system for rating clinical guidelines. PLoS Med 2009; 6:e1000094.
20. Mayer D. Applicability and strength of evidence. In: Mayer D, editor. Essential evidence-based medicine. 2nd edition. New York: Cambridge University Press; 2010. p. 187–98.
21. Joanna Briggs Institute. The JBI approach. South Australia (AU): University of Adelaide; 2014. Available at: http://joannabriggs.org/jbi-approach.html. Accessed October 2, 2016.
22. Schünemann H, Brozek J, Guyatt G, et al. GRADE handbook. Hamilton, Ontario, Canada: McMaster University; 2013. Available at: http://gdt.guidelinedevelopment.org/central_prod/_design/client/handbook/handbook.html. Accessed October 15, 2016.
23. Berkman ND, Lohr KN, Ansari M, et al. Grading the strength of a body of evidence when assessing health care interventions for the Effective Health Care Program of the Agency for Healthcare Research and Quality: an update. Rockville (MD): Agency for Healthcare Research and Quality, Effective Health Care Program; 2013. Available at: https://effectivehealthcare.ahrq.gov/search-for-guides-reviews-and-reports/?pageaction=d. Accessed October 16, 2016.
24. LeFevre ML, Siu AL, Bibbins-Domingo K. The guide to clinical preventive services, 2014: recommendations of the U.S. Preventive Services Task Force. Rockville (MD): Information for Health Professionals, US Preventive Services Task Force; 2014. Available at: https://www.uspreventiveservicestaskforce.org/Page/Name/tools-and-resources-for-better-preventive-care. Accessed October 2, 2016.
25. Younger P. Internet-based information-seeking behaviour amongst doctors and nurses: a short review of the literature. Health Info Libr J 2010;27:2–10.
26. Gardois P, Calabrese R, Colombi N, et al. Effectiveness of bibliographic searches performed by paediatric residents and interns assisted by librarians: a randomized controlled trial. Health Info Libr J 2011;28:273–84.

The Lived Experience of Anemia Without a Cause

Patricia O'Malley, PhD, RN, APRN-CNS[a,b,*]

KEYWORDS

- Anemia • Pernicious anemia • Anemia without bleeding • Autoimmune disease
- Vitamin B12 therapy • Iron therapy • Sadness

KEY POINTS

- Anemia symptom burden is significant outside and inside the intensive care unit.
- Diagnosis of anemia without bleeding is complex.
- Pernicious anemia has an insidious onset with slow progress and affects the hematologic, gastrointestinal, and neurologic systems.
- Failure to recognize and treat pernicious anemia can result in permanent cognitive and/or motor impairments.

AUTHOR'S NOTE TO THE READER

Evidence has become the mantra for twenty-first century health care. Nurses practice in a sea of evidence in every setting, every day. Evidence has become the final metric for nearly all aspects of nursing care: practice, patient outcomes, evaluation, and education. Often it seems that the most valuable evidence comes only from clinical trials, publications, or well-powered statistical findings.

Evidence describing the suffering associated with anemia from a patient experience is slim. This article is an attempt to integrate *the evidence* and *the experience* of anemia of one patient. Before each section of this review are the words of the patient living with anemia while trying to find a diagnosis. Not every cause of anemia is explored in this article. This patient's experience described here is not every patient's experience.

However, this author hopes that *the integration of experience and evidence in this case* may provide the clinician a broader perspective when caring for persons with anemia. May the anemic patient under your care find understanding, compassion, and hope in the darkness and fatigue.

---

[a] Department of Nursing Research, Premier Health, Center of Nursing Excellence, 1 Wyoming Street, Dayton, OH 45409, USA; [b] School of Nursing, Indiana University East, 2325 Chester Boulevard, Richmond, IN 47374, USA
* Department of Nursing Research, Premier Health, Center of Nursing Excellence, 1 Wyoming Street, Dayton, OH 45409.
E-mail address: pomalley@premierhealth.com

Crit Care Nurs Clin N Am 29 (2017) 389–396
http://dx.doi.org/10.1016/j.cnc.2017.04.007
0899-5885/17/© 2017 Elsevier Inc. All rights reserved.
ccnursing.theclinics.com

A feeling of sadness and longing
That is not akin to pain,
And resembles sorrow only
As the mist resembles the rain.[1]

Darkness is my closest friend.

—*Psalm 88:18 NIV*

DECEMBER

Subjective: In the midst of celebrations, strangely sad. There are no reasons to be so deeply sad. I feel guilty for feeling sad. Guilt doesn't make the sadness less. Sad never goes away. Sad is dark. Sad is scary. Maybe sad is holiday stress.
Objective: Family physician evaluation.
Assessment: Negative examination. Negative laboratory tests.
Plan: Sad will pass. Take some time off.

Evidence

In a survey of 889 patients registered with a pernicious anemia (PA) support group, one-third of patients reported symptoms for 1 year before diagnosis. Fourteen percent reported waiting more than 10 years before receiving a correct diagnosis and treatment. Patients reported memory loss (78%), poor concentration (79%), emotional lability (86%), and suicidal ideation (22%) before treatment.[2] Because a PA diagnosis is a complex process, detection is often missed. As a result, prevalence is probably underestimated.[3] Not all patients with PA display macrocytic red blood cell (RBC) indices. Usually the masking of macrocytosis is the result of a coexistent cause of microcytosis, such as iron deficiency or thalassemia trait. PA has an insidious onset with slow progress and affects the hematologic, gastrointestinal (GI), and neurologic systems.[4]

MARCH

Subjective: Winter goes on and on. Sad has brought fatigue along to stay. No energy. Less and less attention to details. No focus. Just getting the work done on the endless checklist is incredible labor. I used to love my work. Why are statistics so hard all of a sudden? I barely get through the day. I forget a lot! Something is really wrong… I have nothing ready for the holiday. So many lists of things to do. I can't keep track of everything anymore. I need more sleep. I wake up tired….all the time. Almost fell yesterday.
Objective: Thyroid tests for annual monitoring of autoimmune thyroid disease.
Assessment: Laboratory tests normal. Probably seasonal affective disorder and stress. Aging takes work!
Plan: Increase activity. Increase Vitamin D. More light. Take a vacation.

Evidence

The most frequent diagnoses before final diagnosis of PA include anxiety, depression, followed by chronic fatigue syndrome, irritable bowel syndrome, hypothyroidism, multiple sclerosis, hypochondria, fibromyalgia, celiac disease, menopause, and diabetes. In a sample of 889 patients, 98% reported a range of neurologic symptoms, including memory loss (78%), poor concentration (75%), clumsiness (66%), pins and needles (66%), poor sleep (64%), confusion (62%), dizziness (59%), headache (52%), word finding difficulty (50%), balance issues (48%), burning feet (33%), and vertigo (33%).[2] PA is strongly associated with depression, mania, and psychosis.[5]

JUNE

Subjective: Vacation. Sad came with me. Perhaps I can leave sad here when I leave. Second day of vacation, began very light postmenopausal bleeding.

Objective: Sad and anxious. My color is so pale. Balance is way off. Can't walk a straight line sometimes. Bumping into walls.

Assessment: First vaginal bleeding since 2004. Gynecologic examination: possible small fibroid.

Plan: Dilation and curettage (D&C) with biopsy. Rule out uterine cancer.

Evidence

Recent evidence suggests that patient history is of little value for predicting the presence of uterine abnormality in women with abnormal bleeding. In premenopausal women, benign lesions are often the cause, and the prevalence of fibroids and polyps increases with advancing age. However, after menopause, the risk of endometrial cancer increases with advancing age.[6]

JULY

Subjective: Maybe I have been sad because of uterine cancer? I should be afraid, but I am just numb. Just numb.

Objective: D&C negative for endometrial cancer.

Assessment: The CRNA (certified registered nurse anesthetist) tells me in the recovery room my preoperative hemoglobin was 8.8! How can this be? I tell her and then the physician that there is no way I bled enough to drop my hemoglobin to 8.8! Where has all my blood gone?

Plan: Referral to gastroenterologist for workup; Rule out GI malignancy.

Evidence

Anemia with iron deficiency without overt GI bleeding suggests cancer in the GI tract. Benign GI causes of anemia include iron malabsorption related to atrophic gastritis, celiac disease, chronic inflammation, and bariatric surgery or chronic bleeding due to ulcers. For unexplained anemia with iron deficiency, serologic celiac disease screening with transglutaminase antibody (immunoglobulin A [IgA] type) and IgA testing is suggested with bidirectional endoscopy (gastroscopy and colonoscopy). Generally, bidirectional endoscopy is not required in premenopausal women less than 40 years of age. Small intestine examination via capsule endoscopy, computed tomography scan, or MRI is not recommended routinely with a negative bidirectional endoscopy. However, these examinations should be considered if signs of inflammatory or malignant small bowel disease are present. Suspicious signs include unplanned weight loss, belly pain, or increasing level of C-reactive protein.[7]

AUGUST

Subjective: Exhausted. I wake up thinking how long before I can go back to bed. My tongue is so sore. I should be happy the GI evaluation is negative. But I feel nothing but sad. No energy. Overwhelming apathy. I don't see as well anymore. Someone must know what is wrong with me! How did this happen to me?

Objective: Endoscopic evaluation negative for malignancy.

Assessment: Hemoglobin falling, low serum ferritin, low serum cobalamin.

Plan: Hematology consult.

Evidence

"You have pernicious anemia. Your body can't make enough working red blood cells because you do not have enough vitamin B12. Because of the B12 deficiency, your red blood cells don't divide normally and are too large. As a result, your tissues and organs do not receive enough oxygen. This is why you are weak, numb, tired, and have trouble walking.... You also have iron deficiency anemia which contributes to the severity of your cognitive symptoms." *In office discussion with hematologist.*

PA is a disease with complex hematologic, gastric, and immunologic elements. Incidence increases with age with highest prevalence in Northern Europeans—especially in the United Kingdom and Scandinavia, and is found in all ethnic groups.[3]

A water-soluble vitamin, B12 (cobalamin) is essential for cellular function produced by microorganisms and available as dietary animal proteins. The average western diet has 5 to 7 μg/d of B12, which is sufficient for metabolic activity. Once vitamin B12 is fully stored in the liver, B12 deficiency occurs in 6 to 12 months after lack of intake or decline in absorption.[8,9] Uptake of B12 is dependent on intrinsic factor (IF) manufactured by gastric parietal cells.[9]

Proteolysis in the stomach releases B12 from food protein. Once released, B12 binds to R-proteins in gastric juice. IF produced by the parietal cells of the stomach travel with the bound B12 to the duodenum. Pancreatic enzymes degrade the R-proteins, which allows the transfer of B12 to IF. Then the IF-B12 moves to the ileum, where it binds to IF-B12 receptors on ileal cells. Ultimately, the process supplies B12 to systemic circulation for activity in lipid, carbohydrate, and protein metabolism and provides critical activity within the Krebs cycle.[4,8]

PA is more often an autoimmune event, which results in atrophy of the gastric mucosa. As a result, the number of parietal cells that produce the IF necessary for B12 absorption is reduced. Erythropoiesis and myelin synthesis decline, which results in megaloblastic anemia, and demyelinating neurologic disease, which will be permanent if not treated.[3,4,8] Early diagnosis and treatment of vitamin B12 deficiency can prevent bone marrow failure and demyelinating peripheral and central nervous system disease.[9,10]

Also implicated in B12 deficiency is atrophic gastritis (also known as type A or type B gastritis), a process of chronic inflammation of the stomach mucosa, leading to loss of gastric glandular cells and their eventual replacement by intestinal and fibrous tissues. As a result, the stomach's secretion of essential substances, such as hydrochloric acid, pepsin, and IF, is impaired, leading to digestive problems and/or vitamin B12 deficiency. Often, this results in megaloblastic anemia with malabsorption of iron, leading to iron deficiency anemia.[1,4] Type A gastritis primarily affects the body/fundus of the stomach and is more common with PA. Atrophic gastritis can be the result of persistent infection with *Helicobacter pylori* or can be autoimmune in origin. Persons with the autoimmune type of atrophic gastritis are at higher risk for gastric carcinoma and achlorhydria.[1,4]

Increasing motor symptoms such as trouble walking is the function of slow dorsal and lateral spinal column degeneration. Demyelination will progress to axonal degeneration and neuronal death if PA is untreated. Mental disturbances can range from forgetfulness to psychosis. Prevalence is more frequent in persons with Grave disease, myxedema, thyroiditis, adrenal insufficiency, and hypoparathyroidism.[3]

Although the most common cause of B12 deficiency is PA, other causes of B12 deficiency include burns, severe trauma, continuous renal replacement therapy, postoperative gastric surgery, small bowel disease, pancreatic disease, as well as the use of proton pump inhibitors (PPIs), metformin, and angiotensin-converting-enzyme inhibitors.[8] Other risks include radiation injury, Crohn disease, parasites, obstructive jaundice, and vegan diet.[9] Also implicated is severe malnutrition, and gastritis of alcohol abuse that leads to acid and pepsin deficiency necessary to liberate B12 from food.[2,8,10,11]

Vitamin B12 excess is associated with renal failure, cancer, leukemia, polycythemia vera, liver disease, and liver cancer. There is no "gold standard" for measuring B12.[8] High serum levels of B12 may also be related to inflammation and a possible independent marker for patient outcomes in the intensive care unit.[12,13]

Laboratory indices for PA include reticulocyte count and hemoglobin (<13 g/dL for men and <12 g/dL for women). RBC's mean corpuscular volume is >120 fL with low levels of serum vitamin B12.[3] However, with nearly 50% false positive or false negative results, and the fact that many patients can have low B12 levels without clinical evidence of B12 deficiency, clinical assessment with measurements of methylmalonic acid or total homocysteine or both may be more useful for those who have not received treatment. Elevated methylmalonic acid, homocysteine, or both can help confirm vitamin B12 deficiency in untreated patients.[9] Patients with positive anti-IF, or antiparietal cell antibodies, should be screened for autoimmune thyroid disease. More than 90% of patients with PA have serum antibodies against gastric parietal cells, and 50% have antibodies against IF.[11] Elevated fasting serum gastrin level and low serum pepsinogen suggest chronic atrophic gastritis and endoscopy may be indicated to screen for gastric cancers and to confirm gastritis.[9]

SEPTEMBER AND OCTOBER

Subjective: Exhausted. Apathetic. Zero energy. Tearful. Lost.
Objective: Pernicious anemia and iron deficiency anemia.
Assessment: Low blood pressure, pallor, edema.
Plan: Weekly cobalamin and iron infusions to begin.

Evidence

Iron deficiency is a known complication of achlorhydria (absent or low production of hydrochloric acid) and may precede the development of PA because an acidic pH facilitates absorption of iron.[14]

In a study of 160 patients with autoimmune gastritis identified by hypergastrinemia and strongly positive antiparietal antibodies, the overlap between 83 subjects presenting with iron deficiency anemia (IDA), 48 with normocytic indices, and 29 with macrocytic anemia was examined. Compared with macrocytic patients, patients with IDA were younger and mostly women. All groups had a high prevalence of thyroid disease (20%) and diabetes (8%), which suggested autoimmune polyendocrine syndrome. The prevalence of H pylori infection was 87.5% at age younger than 20 years, 47% at age 20 to 40 years, 37.5% at 41 to 60 years, and 12.5% at age older than 60 years. These findings suggest that PA is not just a disease of aging, and that PA may begin many years before clinical symptoms by an autoimmune process most likely started by H pylori.[14]

Conventional diagnostic workups fail to establish the cause of iron deficiency in about a third of patients, and causes of iron deficiency vary by stages of life, gender, and socioeconomic circumstances. Although dietary sources of iron are important, IDA is commonly attributed to blood loss associated with occult bleeding from the GI tract due to malignancy. Increasing availability of noninvasive screening tools to identify celiac disease, autoimmune atrophic gastritis, and H pylori infection has greatly facilitated more precise diagnosis and treatment of IDA.[14]

Iron is an essential element for biological activities, including respiration, energy creation, and DNA production. Iron is stored in the body through breakdown and recycling of red cells. The recycling of aging erythrocytes through phagocytosis by macrophages takes place under the direction of the peptide hormone hepcidin, which is synthesized in the liver.[15]

Iron deficiency or reduction of iron stores is a top-ranking cause of anemia worldwide, which results in microcytic hypochromic red cells. Iron deficiency can be related to increased demand (infancy, menstrual blood loss, pregnancy, blood donation), environmental (diet, poverty), disease (decreased absorption or chronic blood loss), drug therapy (glucocorticoids, salicylates, nonsteroidal anti-inflammatory drugs, PPI), genetics, treatment with erythropoiesis-stimulating drugs, and chronic kidney disease.[15]

However, most cases of IDA are related to GI abnormality. Bariatric surgery has been implicated to removal of iron absorption sites from GI tract and increased gastric pH after surgery. Emerging evidence of H pylori antibodies directed against epitopes on gastric mucosal cells in atrophic gastritis further supports the theory of autoimmune processes triggered by H pylori through antigenic mimicry.[14,15]

Patients with IDA experience weakness, fatigue, difficulty concentrating, and poor work productivity related to low delivery of oxygen and decreased activity of iron-based enzymes. Laboratory serum ferritin is the most sensitive and specific test for iron deficiency (<30 μg/L), and levels can be even lower with anemia. Transferrin saturation level (<16%) suggests the iron supply is insufficient for erythropoiesis. For persons with evidence of inflammation, heart failure, or kidney disease, diagnosis of IDA should rely more on assessment and symptom burden than blood test results. Patients with severe IDA with heart failure or angina should be given an RBC infusion to correct hypoxia because 1 unit of RBC supplies about 200 mg of iron.[15]

NOVEMBER TO MAY

Subjective: The first iron infusion was light! I left the treatment area feeling different. One day after the first infusion, sad began to leave my soul. I am alive again! By the fourth infusion, sad left as quietly as it came. What gift to wake up and not feel sad. Energy returned with every infusion and B12 injection. Able to do math again! I can walk a straight line! My balance is back!

Objective: Blood pressure back to baseline, laboratory tests normal, color pink, no peripheral edema.

Assessment: Balance significantly improved, requiring less sleep. Mood significantly improved.

Plan: Lifelong monitoring. Monthly cobalamin therapy. Iron infusions as needed.

Evidence

Two-thirds of iron is bound to hemoglobin in an adult, with the remaining iron stored in ferritin in all types of cells. Only a few milligrams actively circulate bound to transferrin. Only iron uptake is regulated because there is no excretion process.[16]

Oral iron replacement is slow, and absorption is usually limited if not impossible in PA. Patients refractory to oral iron therapy should be evaluated for autoimmune gastritis. Loss of parietal cells reduces secretion of gastric acid required to absorb iron, which usually precedes vitamin B12 deficiency.[16] Intravenous iron provides more rapid restoration of iron stores. Ferritin levels should be considered 8 to 12 weeks after treatment when results more closely reflect actual iron stores.[17] Patients will require lifetime monitoring for IDA and vitamin B12 deficiency.

Intravenous iron infusions require monitoring. Side effects can include nausea, vomiting, pruritus, headache, flushing, myalgia, joint pain, and back and chest pain, which usually resolve within 48 hours. Hypersensitivity is a rare event.[15] As for vitamin B12 replacement, intramuscular cyanocobalamin (US) and hydroxocobalamin (Europe) injection, about 10% of the injected dose is retained. Doses can be provided up to several times a week until improvement in symptoms and then monthly.

Reticulocyte counts usually increase the first week, and megaloblastic anemia can be corrected in 6 to 8 weeks. Neurologic symptoms subside slowly, weeks to months based on the severity and duration of symptoms before treatment – usually within 6 months.[9]

Post script

A fatal form of anemia with gastric degeneration was first described in 1824 by J.S. Combe in Edinburgh and later by Dr Thomas Addison in 1849. Anton Biermer labeled this fatal disorder in 1872 pernicious anemia.[2,3]

PA was fatal until 1926, when physicians Minot and Murphy described the use of liver to "cure" PA.[2] By 1934, an estimated 15 to 20,000 lives were saved by the treatment diet of liver, leafy vegetables, fruit, eggs, and milk. This diet rich in iron and purine derivatives increased reticulocyte counts and hemoglobin. George Minot (1885–1950) and anemia studies physicians (William P. Murphy [1892–1987] and George H. Whipple [1878–1976]) were the first Americans to receive the Nobel Prize (1934) in physiology or medicine for their work.[18,19]

The vast role of vitamin B12 in metabolism and the treatment of B12 deficiency was uncovered slowly. The next scientific advance was made by William Castle (1897–1990), who discovered the gastric link identified as IF missing in PA and first described the pathophysiology of PA. In 1960, Michael Schwartz demonstrated that patients with PA had antibodies against IF.[3] In 1962, James Irvine identified the presence of additional autoantibodies against parietal cells in stomach mucosa.[3,20,21] Finally, Dorothy Hodgkin's work in identifying the structure of vitamin B12 and insulin brought her the Nobel Prize in 1964.[18]

Patients that complain of a "strange tiredness" or waking up exhausted with cognitive and motor issues should trigger suspicion of PA and/or IDA especially if there is history of autoimmune thyroid disease.[2] Of course, GI malignancy must be ruled out. However, treatment of PA can begin while determining any other causal factors.

Insidious and dark, PA can be identified EARLY by listening to the patient's description of how they are doing mentally, physically, and spiritually. One way to begin an assessment is to ask, *"Is there anything I should know that you have not told me?"*

REFERENCES

1. Henry Wadsworth Longfellow (1807-1882). The Day is Done. 1844. Available at: https://www.poetryfoundation.org/poems-and-poets/poets/detail/henry-wadsworth-longfellow. Accessed December 30, 2016.

2. Hooper M, Hudson P, Porter F, et al. Patient journeys: diagnosis and treatment of pernicious anaemia. Br J Nurs 2014;23(7):376–81.
3. Bizzaro N, Antico A. Diagnosis and classification of pernicious anemia. Autoimmun Rev 2014;13(4–5):565–8.
4. Green R. Anemias beyond B12 and iron deficiency: the buzz about other B's, elementary and nonelementary problems. Hematol Am Soc Hematol Educ Program 2012;2012:492–8. Available at: http://asheducationbook.hematologylibrary.org/content/2012/1/492.long. Accessed November 26, 2016.
5. Bram D, Bubrovszky M, Durand JP, et al. Pernicious anemia presenting as catatonia: correlating vitamin B12 levels and catatonic symptoms. Gen Hosp Psychiatry 2015;37(3):273.e5-7.
6. Van den Bosch T, Ameye L, Van SchouBroeck D, et al. Intra-cavitary uterine pathology in women with abnormal uterine bleeding: a prospective study of 1220 women. Facts Views Vis Obgyn 2015;7(1):17–24.
7. Dahlerup JF, Eivindson M, Jacobsen BA, et al. Diagnosis and treatment of unexplained anemia with iron deficiency without overt bleeding. Dan Med J 2015; 62(4):C5072.
8. Romain M, Sviri S, Linton DM, et al. The role of vitamin B12 in the critically ill- a review. Anaesth Intensive Care 2016;44(4):447–52.
9. Stabler SP. Vitamin B12 deficiency. N Engl J Med 2013;368(2):149–60.
10. Shipton MJ, Thachil J. Vitamin B12 deficiency- a 21st century perspective. Clin Med 2015;15(2):145–50.
11. Bunn HF. Vitamin B12 and pernicious anemia- the dawn of molecular medicine. N Engl J Med 2014;370(8):773–6.
12. Sviri S, Khalaila R, Daher S, et al. Increased vitamin B12 levels are associated with mortality in critically ill medical patients. Clin Nutr 2012;31(1):53–9.
13. Hershko C, Ronson A, Souroujon M, et al. Variable hematologic presentation of autoimmune gastritis: age-related progression from iron deficiency to cobalamin depletion. Blood 2006;107(4):1673–9.
14. Hershko C, Skikne B. Pathogenesis and management of iron deficiency anemia: emerging role of celiac disease, Helicobacter pylori, and autoimmune gastritis. Semin Hematol 2009;46(4):339–50.
15. Camaschella C. Iron-deficiency anemia. N Engl J Med 2015;372(19):1832–43.
16. Kulnigg-Dabsch S. Autoimmune gastritis. Wien Med Wochenschr 2016; 166(13–14):424–30.
17. Jimenez K, Kulnigg-Dabsch S, Gasche C. Management of iron deficiency anemia. Gastroenterol Hepatol 2015;11(4):241–50.
18. Scott JM, Molloy AM. The discovery of vitamin B12. Ann Nutr Metab 2012;61(3): 239–45.
19. Kyle RA, Shampo MA. George R. Minot- Nobel Prize for the treatment of pernicious anemia. Mayo Clin Proc 2002;77(11):1150.
20. Irvine WJ. Immunologic aspects of pernicious anemia. N Engl J Med 1965;273: 432–8.
21. Irvine WJ. The association of atrophic gastritis with autoimmune thyroid disease. Clin Endocrin Metab 1975;4(2):351–77.

Printed and bound by CPI Group (UK) Ltd, Croydon, CR0 4YY

03/10/2024

01040390-0008